the new rules of wellness

Transformational Stories from Health
Experts Who Lead from the Heart

House of Wellness Publishing

HOUSE OF WELLNESS
PUBLISHING

Disclaimer

All the information, techniques, skills, and concepts contained within this publication are of the nature of general comment only and are not in any way recommended as individual advice. The intent is to offer a variety of information to provide a wider range of choices now and in the future, recognising that we all have widely diverse circumstances and viewpoints. Should any reader choose to make use of the information contained herein, this is their decision and the author and publishers do not assume any responsibilities whatsoever under any condition or circumstances.

-WW→

Foreword by Dr. Dee Hacking

When loss, change, and a new direction are inevitable, look at 'what is' and not 'what was,' and start to think and feel about the energy behind WHAT IF and WHAT CAN BE.

Rain is the white noise of nature. Panic is the not-so-static white noise of overwhelm.

I watched intently as the pearly droplets chased each other down the porthole window, my mind using them as an escape from the confined reality of this small cabin. The seats resemble bespoke van upholstery. I know an uncomfortable chair can be critical on longer flights, but this will be a short one to a remote Victorian destination for aeromedical services. Sitting on the runway at Essendon Airport feeling clammy and nauseous from the instant, unexpected bout of claustrophobia, the Royal Flying Doctor Service fixed-wing Twin Turbo King Air B350C whirled her propellers, and the cabin shuddered.

I wanted to be taking charge in the pilot seat wearing the crisp white shirt with the bars and wings next to my co-pilot, but that dream would be unrealized. My career as a Physician in the RFDS was also over then - I passed out as we took off. The cabin space closed in on me, and that white noise filled the compartment; the last thing I recalled was the nurse touching my flushed cheeks; I guess I became the first patient that day.

Why am I sharing this with you?

Because sometimes life gets in the way of a plan, and it's okay to segway into something else. I have worked with thousands over the past 30 years in my Allied Health business in clinical settings and with my writing and publishing, assisting them along their creative journey, health, and injury management journeys when life has struck them down. And now helping others realize their dreams of becoming published authors. When they needed the inspiration to know where to start when they felt overwhelmed or stuck, a byproduct of conversation and stories is the influence we share valuable insight 'without being told' by becoming inspired by what others are doing; to simply *gain a solution inside inspiration, and to feel healthy!* Health is a state of body, mind, and social wellness; it's multi-dimensional and encourages a balanced state of practicing habits regularly to train physical and mental outcomes so that instead of just surviving, you're thriving—dimensions of mental, physical, social, financial, spiritual, environmental, and vocational. *I now go beyond other people's fears and limitations and* assist others to do the same.

I also had one of my biggest challenges where I lost my confidence, passion, health, and motivation to keep going. My life fell apart. I lay in my bed for three days in the fetal position, my kids having to fend for themselves, it seemed, at the time. (I did have help; they weren't defenseless, they were of double-digit ages, and I was the defenseless one).

A client of mine sat in her car out the front of our house after injuring herself at beach boot camp at sunrise. "I know you are in there," she shouted. I pulled myself out of bed, horrified; it was 0600, but this exact moment was the push I needed. She told me stories about her life and how she was trying to survive, and I listened. (She was unaware of my 'survival mode,' of course). She then continued and referenced that if I don't 'fix *her body, she can't work.*' Over the next twenty minutes, I intently got to fixing and remedying her buckled ankle so she could walk.

"OK, off to work for me"! she said as if the shout-at-the-window-from-the-front-street event hadn't occurred. "Thank You so much; my life depends on you, Dee; our whole family does; don't you go anywhere, will you!" Sharon said.

I, too, picked up my game and found myself back to living well and moving forward, no matter what. The byproduct of that conversation and addressing my purpose pushed my life troubles aside, and found a way to become happy again. It is "my" mind that creates my experiences. We are all unlimited in our ability to make the good in life.

Trajectories appear and manifest change that leads you on a more significant path that will serve you better than you ever imagined. Be like the arrow, strike your mark, always moving forwards. It takes just one story, action, or sometimes comment to *repair* what seems irreparable.

That day with the RFDS, those years ago, when I recovered from the flight, I knew whatever I did in the future, I would support the Royal Flying Doctor Service, which I have done for the past 30 years. In addition, the profits of the e-book/kindle version of this series will be donated to my passionate cause, keeping the vital aeromedical service in the air, looking after regional Australians and emergency transport services. I could not directly be involved, and my pilot career was also over, and I'm now OK with all of that and striking forward in all that I do.

In life, white noise is all around us. It can silence us or propel us. Life offers adversity, overwhelming challenges, emotional triggers, and what may feel like a dead-end health crisis. Yet, l along these pathways, we must be traveling within our journeys gives us all opportunities to invent new rules to traverse life, navigate our wellness and our businesses, and find practices and tips that suit us best. The golden moments lie within the sharing of these stories creating change and saving the lives of others. To heal ourselves and communicate profound messages from our hearts is an energetic vision that inspires me daily to do all I do.

Within The New Rules of Wellness, volume 1 of the book series, you will hear from a cross-section of professionals with different approaches, insight from their health journeys, and professional experiences that have inspired the desire to serve others, offering enrichment. You create your wellness by addressing the big-picture concepts about the health industry, addressing the need for many shifts and total revolution in some areas caring about the happiness of others.

My passionate desire to offer the opportunity to share The New Rules of Wellness Volume 1 in the space of health with expert knowledge via stories from extraordinary individuals and health experts and professionals that lead from the heart in all that they do, was realized this year.

You will read about many inspirational authors sharing transformational stories rising above all the white noise and creating refreshing new rules around health and wellness, becoming visionaries within their businesses, and communicating with you timeless advice while shining irreplaceable light into enhancing others' journeys.

Your wellness starts with you! Creating the life you want to live begins with you.

New rules also start with you! Inspiration is around if you edit the white noise out and become centered.

Dr. Dee Hacking
Ph.D.BHMS.B.Sc.Adv.Dip.Hom.Adv.Dip.RT

Founder, Doctor, Homoeopathic Physician, Coach, Author, and Publisher.

House of Wellness Publishing

Your story, too, is waiting to be told! Ready to write a book? Reach out, and I can make that happen.

Email: houseofwellnesspublishing@gmail.com
LinkedIn: www.linkedin.com/n/Dr. Dee Middendorp-Hacking
Facebook: www.facebook.com/houseofwellnesspublishing

Contents

-vW→

Dr. Dee Hacking

Abundance starts with contentment.

ABBA played on the Automatic-Phillips record player turntable, now a beautiful piece of antique furniture that was considered at the time of production in the '70s to be a remarkable piece of technology. I watched the needle pick up the groove on the Vinyl LP.

'I DO I DO I DO I DO,' I sing along, followed by *'Rock Me'* on side B.

I inspected the classic album cover and admired the well-dressed quartet in the back seat of a vintage vehicle sipping champagne from silver goblets. I flicked the LP to side A, and *'Mamma Mia'* began. I was so inspired that I got to work on the art pieces I was commissioned to complete along with my Biology and English literature homework, and I completed everything in hours. I accomplished so much that day at home in 1988; I was 15 years old and was inspired.

Now that I'm approaching fifty, my first personal rule of wellness has not changed; Feel inspired and ready to take action, and the desired result automatically follows with a strict deadline in place.

To this day, music is one of my primary motivators, and Bjorn, Freda, Benny, and Agnatha still sing to me, but from my desktop. ABBA sang to me throughout my schooling and University studies for seventeen years. Now, I play a song each morning as I set up for my clinical day as a Homeopathic Physician, Injury management specialist in my home Publishing office.

I sing along inspired, *'I DO I DO I DO I DO'!*

Some days I'm unstoppable, waking up early excited about life, and can't wait to start my day. On other days, I must get off the bed as I'm late for the couch.

Some days are about fun and relationships, others are about business and clinical work, and others are about personal confidence and artistic passions. Yet, days do exist when inspiration is in the lack.

I say to myself, "Dear mind give yourself a break!"

Individual wellness is a version of the self-care wheel for a daily lifestyle application: physical, psychological, emotional, spiritual, personal, and professional arenas. Self-assessment is then needed for accountability with an understanding of one's values, beliefs, and morals. Each of our lives has brought unique circumstances, but the goals seem similar: find what makes us feel our best.

What can we learn? To feel better!

Acknowledging the interconnectedness of mental and physical wellness invites HUGE shifts.

Positive self-reinforcement and finding the excellent feeling within each hour of each day will get you there every time. Recalibrate if needed, don't give up on yourself, and change the plan a little. Having a relationship with yourself, your heart, and your soul (the essence of your being and definitive life purpose). Having a relationship with people around you and relating to your environment and culture. Experiencing life according to your life purpose and caring about it all too.

Abundance starters with contentment, I would love to tell my 15-year-old self this. Send her a letter and tell her to keep singing her ABBA songs as inspiration or whatever pushes her to become contented. This is where the energy of success, purpose, and direction flows. I'm sure we are all searching for that feel-good feeling somewhere; usually, the search is outside ourselves, but it's an inside job. I'd tell her to write her life's song, and she can change the lyrics as often as she likes.

Calm the inner, and life will flow organically.

I had recently decided to go on a week-long retreat. I saw on FaceBook that a colleague had done so, and she spoke of all the transformational events, the soul-enhancing journey, and the enriching internal changes. BRILLIANT, I need that; I set about looking. Most of what I found was unsuitable, so I planned a "retreat day" once a fortnight. I'd wake up and PRETEND I was in a health retreat for the whole day. I made a list of ideas of ALL the possible things one does on a retreat:

Meditation/candle/oils/essential oils on my feet/isopisiform acupressure points
Massage/acupressure /Yoga/Swim/Fitness
Self-care/face mask/hair mask
Float tank/pedicure/reflexology /simple foot soak in a bucket
Spiritual Journey/Reading/Writing/Art/creativity
Connect with nature/disconnect with technology
Visualization /Relaxation/self-connection/self-education/sleep
Nutrition meals/juice fast

No technology, no rushing, no toxins, no overeating, no overwhelm, no stress, no work, no deadlines, no ANYTHING that doesn't serve me well. The truth is that life detoxing requires a holistic approach, not a quick fix—a consistent application.

As I professionally know, a healthy liver naturally cleanses itself; dietary stressors and environmental toxins can get in the way of optimal liver function. Hence, the Liver focus is an excellent dual approach. Making strategic diet and lifestyle shifts can help counter effects, support the liver's detoxification, and lighten our overall toxic load.

SO ADDING ON RETREAT DAY: Fenugreek seeds, Dandelion, Glutathione, Turmeric Vitamin C, and an Activated Charcoal supplementation.

A truly effective and sustainable liver detox/ life detox involves implementing strategic nutrition and lifestyle shifts (tailored supplementation, sweating regularly, managing daily stress, and adopting a liver-friendly diet). Intermittent fasting is your body's chance to leave work and catch up on house cleaning! Schedule a daily sweat session. Practice self-care to optimize mental and physical well-being; it's in your best interest to address unchecked stress and adopt healthy habits that promote a calm, happy life. Something as simple as an aromatherapy bath or foot soak once or twice a week can do the trick on busy working weeks. I was excited to start.

Retreat Day arrived:

I wake up before sunrise, do sunrise yoga on my balcony, freshly squeezed vegetable juice breakfast and essential oils, and meditate. Stationary bike ride at our apartment complex gym, a swim in our pool, and a sweat session. Lunch is a small carrot/apple/celery juice. A magnesium float tank session and massage, finishing the day with a light protein meal with dark leafy greens. Snuggling up for a cuddle with hubby and herbal tea on the couch, early to bed to read, meditate, then have a good night's sleep.

My New Rule of Wellness: Non-negotiable Retreat Day!

I've set aside two months, TWO CONSECUTIVE RETREAT DAYS! Double Bliss!

The magnesium float session triggered a memory I didn't know existed.

I entered the dimly lit Spa room and indulged in the pre-float shower. Outstanding Lemon Myrtle/ sugar body scrub, my whole body felt like silk. Like the water in the Cocoon movie, the float tank water was glowing blue.

My immersed body floated in the warm water, my hair moving around me in the tiny currents of my slight hand movements, lid open. The music piped in, I couldn't recall where I had heard the song before. I closed my eyes, allowing the water to support me, and I was catapulted back to 1988. I was 15 again, floating in a tank similar to this one. I could hear my Mother asking if I was alright; she was also in a tank. I answered her and noticed what looked like a million stars around me. Felt like I was floating in the Universe. All the tension evaporated from my body, and I heard that same song today. I can feel the magnesium sulfate passing directly into my tissues, and I think a cellular energy connection. I also feel my skin tingling, and I know my inner regeneration and repair mechanisms are fired into action, increasing the recovery of my joints and muscles. Each cell in my body is communicating with the other cells. I feel now as I felt in the 1988 float.

I had forgotten that ever happened.

The song evoked electric vigor within me. I later found 'Neon Abyss-Retro Wave Ambiance' on YouTube, a set of repeating binaural beats; I now play this each morning after my morning meditation to evoke my inner healing processes.

I'm so glad I went on this 'Retreat' journey of my own accord. My body pain has significantly reduced, my muscles and nerves that were previously numb are activated, my energy levels have increased, digestion and weight loss have been triggered, and I feel relaxed and on purpose.
Q: Is it time to take yourself on a date? A: YES! ...."I DO I DO I DO I DO I DO!!"

"Working on yourself, your health, and wellness amplifies your life and your business, not the other way around."

Working diligently without concern for the results is exactly what brings in the results.

My husband John and I have created a life where we don't wait all week for Friday to arrive to enjoy life; we feel fulfilled and healthy enjoying each day of the week.

My passion and purpose are to focus on my patients in my clinical work, within my writing work, and on the fantastic Authors I work with, supporting them as their publisher and Ghostwriter. Figuring out the remedy to whatever is going on in life and formulating consecutive and compounding steps towards feeling great, happy, and nourished is fulfilling.

Amy is a patient with consultations virtually via Zoom as she resides in another country.

"I'm so stressed about failing and not being healthy that I get myself out of bed to exercise, freak out as my clothes don't fit, and go straight back to bed frozen in my guilt, I hate my life, I hate myself!" - Amy, 2022

"Amy, let's think about it a little bit."

We both have jotting paper and pen.

"You write down what you hate, and I will retort that with an idea, and let's work out a daily life plan you would love to live 6-12 months from now."

She looked at me through the screen, shocked. "Oh, I thought you would prescribe me an antidepressant!"

She wrote.

I waited.

"I hate my body - I'm a failure- I see myself as obese, flabby, with ugly thin hair. I'm lifeless most of the time and unmotivated with no energy, I skip meals trying to lose weight, try every diet, and I want to be energetic in the morning and feel comfortable in my clothing. I need to feel sexy again and have a great intimate relationship with my husband. My ultimate dream is to study and develop new skills in Psychology and open my practice, I stop myself by watching NetFlix, but I never get around to studying. I'm not social, I feel I'm 'fake' and have imposter syndrome, life is hard work that exhausts me, and I just don't enjoy my life, to be fair."

MY RETORT: Let's find an exercise you love and a song that inspires you. Add strength training exercises you can do in the morning before your busy day starts elevating serotonin and endorphin levels - the body's happy chemicals. Let's choose an appropriate breakfast you love, a meal preparation plan to avoid skipping (or quick) meals, targeted nutrition, and portion planning. A focus on your hormone levels homeopathically is needed to address your weight loss, thinning hair, mojo, concentration, stress levels, and mental focus. Let's get a plan together to sign up for an upgrade of your qualifications (there is never a right time to get started, just get started and map out a simple step-by-step action over time to move forward).

Personal accountability often lies within the 'doing' of it; the rest will flow organically. Let's map out a business plan for the new practice. Scheduled downtime is vital to do the things you love, like watching your shows, dates with your husband, socializing, and creative activities - all tools that expand your heart center and increase enjoyment in life.

"GREAT! I love Yoga and swimming, I haven't listened to music for a long time, and I ordered new swimmers and goggles, but they are still in their packets. I wanted to do a Carnivore eating plan but felt unmotivated. My hormones have been imbalanced for years affecting those around me and my mental focus. The course upgrade I need to do that, I have already mapped out a plan for my clinic, but never kept going due to my self-sabotaging thoughts- felt I didn't deserve it. Looking at it, I suppose I had started but never kept going; thank You, Dr. Dee, for the realization and accountability."

THE PLAN: Yoga, swimming, Static Wall Pilates Strength Training program online, breathe-work on a weekly plan, and meditation. Carnivore lifestyle plan with supplementation of Betaine HCL, Magnesium, Vit C, Glycine, and Liver capsules. Ginkgo Biloba for mental focus and Rosemary essential oil to inhale while studying for mental stamina. The homeopathic plan for the hormone imbalance included Sepia, and Amy's Constitutional remedy application is Nux Vomica. 'Netflixing' is kept for after the scheduled study sessions, a non-negotiable date with the husband on the 20th of each month (as that is their wedding anniversary date), and a monthly catchup date with the girlfriends; coffee, pedicure, Paint-and Sip class/ Macrame/ Pottery class, something FUN. Working diligently without concern for the results is precisely what brings in the results, setting up a 'lifestyle that you love' toward the direction that will have the effects naturally flow.

UPDATE: Over 6 months, Amy has lost 2 dress sizes with the inspiration to keep going; her toned body and new clothes have her feeling comfortable in her skin. Her husband loves preparing and cooking on the grill while Amy completes her afternoon study session, loving the eating plan's flexibility and simplicity. She watches her shows as a wind down (no longer as an escape from the world). Amy has nearly completed her practitioner upgrades and has found office space. The excitement is brewing as her husband has suggested they plan to purchase the office and set up their private practice, Chiropractor, and they can work together. Her husband would only have considered his practice with this new lifestyle setup and opportunity.

"The magic has been hidden in the little daily steps. We love our new life, and I love myself, thanks to you, Dr. Dee. My husband and I are so grateful for you co-creating a life we love. We feel fulfilled and

healthy to enjoy daily!" - Amy, March 2023.

I became a DOER and a Self-Believer!

I never found any meaning behind the question, "Can I do this?" Of course, I can, but will I?

Inspiration? YES, for sure. Motivation? Not really, NO.

BUT THERE IS MORE.

Visualizing the result? HELL YES!

FEEL like you've already done it. You've made it. Achieved it. YES!

Lay it all out the night before. So I get up and do it. No thinking, no talking myself out of it. Not letting a spec of fear dwell inside and not letting it take over.

Believe, Believe, Believe.

Whatever you want to do, Believe it - even if you don't believe it.

Play the game of belief, act as if you believe it and have achieved it, and it will happen. That is sheer power - and it will happen. It's worked in my life, and it will work in yours.

Trace connected with me in an application to be featured in my multi-author book series.

"I've always wanted to be a published author; I've written many half-completed projects and never knew the next step." She excitedly explained on the phone. "I'd love to share my work as I'm passionate about making my mark on the world. I want to stand on international stages and help people. I just don't know how to pick the information from my head and write it figuratively and passionately in my story."

"Life is simple and easy if you make it that way with the right assistance!" I replied.

She continued to explain she was looking for an 'energy connection with the right person, telling herself to have more patience and wait for the right writer/publisher to come along when it felt suitable for her.

I explained that all my ventures are fully supported each step of the way, group coaching with connection with other like-minded and like-energy professionals who support each other, meeting recordings to work from, lots of guidance, and lots to assist her in shining and spotlighting her passion and profession, lots of vibes, and buzz. **Let's get you published!**

"I feel that I now flow freely with my thoughts and words. I've let go of all expectations and let the 'flow' happen. I write in a state of peace

and love being included in your book Dr. Dee and look forward to writing more with you and producing my solo book as well. Becoming a published author has not only checked my goal boxes but also provided the knowledge to become the author I have always desired. It has expanded my business, made me stand out in my profession, and has been a valuable marketing tool! I've now been inspired to keep writing and completing my other projects. EXCITING!" - Trace, 2023.

Be the 1% that 99% of others won't be. Reach out to me and see how I can assist you best. This can be the magic of your health and wellness journey via confident, consistent choices and small actions, empowering you to live the life you love, a life you don't need an escape from.

Dr. Nereda (Dee) Hacking
Ph.D.BHMS.B.Sc.Adv, Dip.Hom.Adv.Dip.RT

About the Author

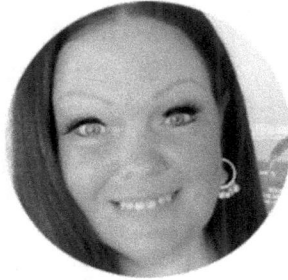

Dr. Dee Hacking is proudly the creator of The New Rules of Wellness book series and is a Publisher, International Bestselling Author, and Ghostwriter in the writing field.

Dee also owns and runs her Allied Health Clinic in Mackay, Australia, where she holds the Homeopathic Physician and Injury Specialist position.

Dr. Dee hails from Metropolitan Melbourne, Australia, and lives in tropical North Queensland, Australia, and the Snowy peaks of Spokane, Washington, USA, with her husband, John Hacking. They are immensely proud to share three adult children and grandchildren, Savannah. When she is not writing in her favorite coffee shop or swimming laps, she curls up in her reading nook.

Email: houseofwellnesspublishing@gmail.com
Facebook: www.facebook.com/nereda.hacking
Instagram: DrDee Hacking (@dr.deehacking) | Instagram

-ww>

Debbie Ahern

Flaming Skies

The flaming orange sky gives way to gentle pinks and mellow golds. The sky seems endless as it spreads out in front of my eyes, I can't help but stare as another day fades, a prelude to the next day, a time to relax and fill my soul with the most beautiful dreams.

Sunsets have always been special to me and offer every cell in my body the chance to recharge. The perfect conclusion to another day in paradise, the one we have created for ourselves over many years. Any resting time, other than the sunsets, was wasting precious time. My husband Mark and I have enjoyed sitting on this fifth-level Mackay Marina balcony witnessing years of pink skies and golden moments. Our career, too, has been golden as business owners of our multiple award-winning and local icon, Debbie's Seafood Superstore, Seafood Vans, and

Debbies Seafood Cafe Mackay from its conception on this same stretch of beach over 30 years ago in the simple aluminum alloy-tinny with a few nets and rods.

We have created all the success we have ever dreamed of. Today our lives changed again with the same magnitude as they did thirty years ago, on the same stretch of Queensland beach.

Empty Oyster shells fall from my plate, tumbling next to the half-empty Merlot bottle, and continue to the tiled floor of our balcony, bringing my attention back to the present moment. I lifted the plate with an unexpected tilt, and more Oyster shells fell as a tear trickled down my cheek. Today, it all happened. The tears, are they of happiness? A tear of sadness, maybe?

No! It's JOY.

Our career has significantly impacted our lives and happiness, and we have achieved a well-lived life. We could go on running our business, yet, who doesn't want to be happier? I don't often ask myself, "Is this all there is?"

ALL THIS, yes, is amazing, but I am constantly curious. I feel like time is slipping me by, I'm not making the most of it now, and I desire to invest in our wealth, a set of new passions. More recently, I have felt that I've compromised my values. An overwhelming sense fills me, the same feeling as *the sky seems endless as it spreads out in front of my eyes, I can't help but stare as another day fades, a prelude to the next day, a time to relax and fill my soul with the most beautiful dreams.*

The following beautiful dream, called life, expands before my eyes, and I'm excited about it.

A farm-girl-tomboy from inland Queensland, I knew all about the harsh heat of summer and the red dust storms. Hard work befalls the land and those who dwell there, and the refined earthy grains of soil get stuck in the corner of your eyes on those summer afternoons accompanied by brilliant sunsets. You would assume I would naturally feel out of place on the water daily in a small Tinny, but I wasn't. Legs sandblasted, chapped salty lips, and the end-of-day exhaustion like no other, but I loved it.

I didn't plan on being a fisherman, but isn't it funny how it works out to be the best thing ever happening when you don't plan something? Despite the sore back, the endless salt sprays to the face, and the lack of hi-tech sounders and charts, one's health I valued as secondary.

Interpreting the ocean, weather forecasting, and the catch quality was first.

The selling of our catch and, later, raising our family. Then, even later, building our business into what it is today. This same stretch of beach where we would haul the small boat up the beach, camp overnight, get eaten alive by the Midges and Mosquitoes, and watch the same magnificent sunsets as the one we witness tonight, making way for brilliant stars and a full moon. It's impressive to note this expansive Marina and high-rise apartment complex over the years mushroomed from 'our fishing beach' and what a place it has been to live.

But this, too, is coming to a close.

'SOLD!' read the sign.

"Shock Decision" the Daily Mercury and The Courier Mail articles read, " After 25 years at the helm of one of Mackay's most popular seafood shops, the founders and their family have decided to put the famous business up for sale".

Messages flooded in.

Some were congratulations, some were good wishes for enjoying retirement, some were reminiscent of the old Salonika beach days, and some were quite shocked, as the title suggests. Some were, "I'm so sorry"!

Media releases and TV interviews followed.

"Debbies Seafood - Mackay's freshest and tastiest is Mackay's largest seafood retailer with roving vans servicing Mackay and the central highlands. After a quarter-century, Debbies is leaving her legacy in somebody else's hands, putting the business on the market and retiring."

"What are you going to do now?" people ask.

"Not sure yet," I replied. "Throw the rocks, and the path shall appear!" This is my New Rule for Wellness. Start, *just start*, to travel along the unknown trajectory and experience the *unfolding*.

A style very unlike me historically.

A determined and strategic organizer with clear, unemotional, and steadfast direction with a work-work-work-till-you-drop persona. *I'm not making the most of now* my body and inner molecules chat together.

Signs appear all over me: what got me here won't get me there!

Where is there? It's exciting along this trajectory; my mitochondria, my cellular powerhouses, now chat and tell me to slow the pace.

Some time ago, I had been sitting on our balcony after my morning Yoga practice; still on my inward journey, the wind picked up and blew some debris off the tiled floor. I witnessed the dried leaf matter float off as it was caught in the gusts and hovered. I blinked.

I double-blinked to focus my gaze, I thought I saw a pathway leading up some invisible stairs; the dry debris made the path appear. Simultaneously a friend's YouTube channel was playing inside our apartment, telling a story from an Indiana Jones movie, 'The Leap of Faith Principle.' The wide ravine may seem very deep in front of you with no way to cross; it's hopeless; you're stuck. Kick, or pick up some rocks and dirt, throw them, and then a pathway shall appear. Place one step before the other - walk - and the path and destination will become more apparent. You don't have to have everything figured out and planned step by step; what a revelation to me!

There had been many moments along our unique life journey and career when I felt exhausted, my body ached, and injuries to the point of blistering and bleeding fingers, hands, and feet. Vertigo, too, had set in, and no time for me, ill health arrived, and there it is, *is this all there is to life?* The downtime was difficult for me. Such a waste of the time I could spend building my business and fishing - *IS THIS IT?* I found myself asking, even in our 'paradise life'?

I sat in my Yoga practice daily feeling unaccomplished, like something was missing from our lives.

Ahhhh, I said to myself. *The matriarch of the business, I think this day has gone; it's run its course. Others' opinions don't matter anymore; time to forge my blissful pathway forward.*

A lump came up in my throat. Sadness or excitement? What lies ahead?

'Who knows' I say out loud and repeat it to myself. *Who Knows!* This emotional journey of late has been the best thing for my knowledge, energy, intuition, and soul purpose.

I feel THIS IS IT! Not IS THIS IT?

Shining and stepping into my power.

Power where every cell in my body listens to each thought I have. My thoughts and actions now serve me well, following a new path, changing life, and evolving. Lots of pushback from some people around me, but I listen to each cell in my body.

My Tomboy self has discovered femininity, and I'm ok with that.

I now SWAN around and enjoy pleasures I had never indulged in before when the business took my time, 80-100 hours each week for years and years; I find I'm doing things for me: Magnesium float tanks, Espresso with friends, social catchups with our daughter and granddaughter, exercise classes together, spending quality time with my Mum and my Sister, poking around and Op-shopping, bare feet in the grass moments, Massages, Yoga courses, Hugs, and retreats, trips to Bali and New Zealand, pedicures...SWANNING...ALL OF IT.

My passion was to build a large business and finally create a passive income.

Tick Tick!

This is a North Queensland saying, Just go with the flow. I now feel like I am. *Go with the flow* is another new rule of wellness for me.

He was the guitar to my string.

Riding horses was my favorite pastime as a child. My father supported all that I did. There is nothing quite like the smell of horse sweat in my nostrils, muscular equine bodies galloping full flight, my hair streaming behind, their manes taking flight, and the thunder of hooves in my ears. I had forgotten about my equine passion in my daily Briny lifestyle, yet the connection with the flora, fauna, and land remains in my heart.

I loved life on the station, riding horses, burying my face in the horse's mane, and inhaling all the smells, and it felt like the entire horse entered my blood system until my neurons vibrated with its essence. The horses' sticky skin, musky ammonia, and latherin aromas are infectious. Being present with all farm animals was my perfect world. When I had a *buster-off-the-horse*, Dad would tell me I owned that patch of earth where I had landed, then encourage me to get back on. I owned many little plots of land in my childhood! We Competed in Gymkhanas & Rodeos, bringing home the occasional trophy or ribbons.

Dad passed years ago, but I still feel a pain in my heart as the memories flood in as I write this. Looking back, I realize how much I loved the Sunday roast dinners with my family—so many special memories.

After several years, we moved to the city, and I never quite gelled. My school teacher, Mr. Esham, asked me what I wanted to do. I replied to attend AG school (Agricultural School) to study Veterinary Science. He so kindly supported me and wrote to the college, and I held my breath, waiting for a reply. I was devastated. 'No, Sorry' was the college's reply. 'Males only.' The facility doesn't cater to Women, I was born 20 years too early.

Another devastating moment that changed me was major heartache in my life.

My first heartbreak was the loss of my sausage dog Cindy. I don't remember, but Dad said I cried myself to sleep for months. When my sister was born several years later, we added Cindy as her second name. One day she said, "You named me after a dog'? I replied, "Yes, but I loved that dog wholeheartedly!" Maybe she didn't quite understand the endearing testament and legacy.

My dad died in 2009, a pivotal point in my life. This huge man wasn't part of it anymore. I remember saying in the hospital room I would gladly change places with him, but his reply was he couldn't do that, with tears streaming down his face. The only time I had ever seen him cry. I would have changed places then and there because I didn't know how to live without him. He was the guitar to my string.

When I play my Ukelele and lightly strum the strings, I feel that Dad owns a patch of my soul.

Balance & Grace

The skies glowed, my eyes closed to rest, and I was one with the stars and the setting sun. I feel every cell in my body communicating with each other. My nervous system is at peace with my endocrine system, the neurons and synapses all chatting and whispering secrets. I feel the connection within me, my connection to my world and the universe.

Before now, I knew my brain's 80 billion nerve cells were of a blocked stimulus. My goal currently is to be balanced. I can easily overwork, overplay, and overachieve. When I'm at the moment I don't release, I may be overdoing it. Maybe I have a superwoman mindset and believe I can do it all until I can't. No one knows what it takes to be me; that is my superpower.

Another new rule of wellness for me is to Rest Purposefully.

I've practiced Yoga for several years but experiencing the benefits of Yoga from a teacher training perspective is a whole new level. Bringing the mind, body, and soul truly together. Feeling the Grace, breathing in the Universe, and breathing out anything that doesn't serve me that I can replace. Spaciousness opens the body, mainly the heart, which many of us protect with copious layers of pearl shell. More Resting —Purposefully.

I now recognize a repeating pattern of ill health.

Balancing physical energy and vitality not to support ME; historically, I supported business and business activities. "Work hard" and "Work till the death" were ideologies of my childhood learnings and family ethics handed down through the generations. Interesting! It doesn't have to be that way, and I know IT IS that way for many people; friends I talk to, family members, and business colleagues. Why do we not tend to support our own health and wellness patterns? Have we lost our way? Most of us haven't, as we sidetracked now and then? Yes, I'd say that's a given in life. Why do we do the opposite of what suits our health and wellness? It may be a 'worthiness' issue or a 'comfort zone issue (I've always done it this way, and it worked, so I keep doing it, change is difficult and often scary). I feel it also may be an 'I'm way down the line of importance, and I run out of time' type of issue.

Deliberate creation versus clarity of balance.

We live in a beautiful time where self-care and access to soulful-stimulating practices are abundant. Benefiting from all this opportunity offers tremendous personal growth, clarity of thoughts, and the realization of self-pressure. Who pressures you the most? Most likely, YOU DO! We bring along all the positive things, and also negative things, from our childhood. We perceive our life from our perspective and bring forth more and more clarity and balance if we allow it, or the opposite effects with the intense stimulation of pressure, which can happen freely and unknowingly. Most of us are distracted by the continuous thought processes that we need the opportunity to develop the balance of our heart center.

Getting back to my gratitude, sitting in my own energetic space. I intend to support others in their Grace and journey, which I now feel is my calling.

Breaking this repeated cycle of ill health, looking beyond myself and my community, to create the intention of being 'less busy,' 'less complicated,' 'less cluttered,' and letting go of my embodying wounds from my past. I recall talking into the mirror a few years ago, I was shocked that I looked so tired. "No more, Debbie!" I repeated to myself, "No More!"

At that point, I didn't have any clue how to start or when to start. When is the right time to begin to look after yourself? Was I selfish? What will others think? All these thoughts track, again, busy brain, but now I feel my soul has lifted from that white noise.

I find it so interesting that what once was vitally important is no longer, and things I used to enjoy I had forgotten about altogether until now; time to FEEL and THINK, and REST.

Instead of trying to EARN abundance and balance, I now ALLOW. Action is nothing to do with abundance. Abundance is a response to my vibration, all those inner cells chatting.

Communicating. Partying. Earning. Allowing.

Whether now or 10 years in the future, all the resources I will ever need are within me, and I have identified that it's my *allowing* the pathway to appear once I start *feeling balanced within Grace.*

What would you do more of if you had all the time and money?

Like most people, I would travel and see the world and explore different cultures, but ultimately I would like to help women and young girls who have been abused. I resonate with the struggle women and young ladies go through in their time of need, abandonment, and abuse. The inner retreating they journey through, the emotional shutdown.

If unsupported, that can be a lifetime struggle of imbalance and negative self-perception. My message would be to savor more and fix less. Laugh more, cry less. You are powerful at creating; nothing is more important than feeling good from the inside out.

I will be successful in all that I do. I own a patch of my soul, a place beautiful dreams grow.

I have always read books to improve myself, usually to improve my self-confidence and build wealth, and now, for fun and it makes me feel great, I love Wilbur Smith's novels about Egypt and listen to audiobooks. Change life up a bit for yourself.

Isn't it funny how it works out to be the best thing ever happening when you don't plan something?

Please connect with me if this resonates with you; I'd love the opportunity to chat. You never know I may be involved with facilitating balance and change with my newly acquired skills.

The next sunset will be even more spectacular, but the unwavering opportunity to rest and connect is still there. Where? I'm still not sure, our new paradise, somewhere blissful.

About the Author

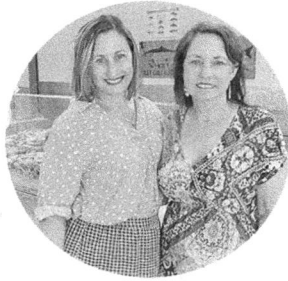

Debbie Ahern, after serving the Greater Mackay region as a local Seafood Icon owning and running Debbies Seafood & Fish Cafe for 3 decades with her husband Mark, and the 'Seafoodie' family, is returning to her natural energy and now writing, becoming a Yoga Teacher, and a Crypto Investor Professional.

At home in Tropical North Queensland, she regularly contributes to her local community and proudly receives many awards. She believes, lives, and breathes daily that Faith, Balance & Grace can change the world.

A lover of Swanning, Art, and Painting, and is most likely the best multi-tasker. You will find her globetrotting, adventuring at a Yoga Retreat, or sipping a Merlot at Sunset. Debbies best advice: Don't be stressed about making waves by being your true self. The moon does it all the time. Just flow freely, embrace the ebb and flow of life.

Email: debbie@debbiesseafood.com.au
LinkedIn: Debbie Ahern

-⌁⟶

Ally Cashen

Rebounding.

I jump fast, I jump slow. I am ready to instruct with the low-impact jogging, the fun dance-inspired cardio routines, and the high-energy bounce interval training as a PT. But my heart is pounding in my chest, not from the aerobic workout I am about to instruct, but from nervousness. My palms are sweaty, and I can hear the mini-trampoline springs squeak a little as I bounce, but that is not what I am concentrating on. The excitement in my chest nearly cuts off my breath; all I have been working on in my personal life and business –is crescendoing to this very moment. Earlier, before the class started, as the new owner of Boogie Bounce Mackay and a newly qualified Bounce instructor, I had briefed my class on safety tips and the health benefits of my fun Bouncing Rebounder Workout, then energetically called out, "LET'S GET JIGGY!"

My whole world stood still just minutes before my commencement exclamation in that class. I felt like I was a deer in headlights. Frozen. Alone. Panicky.

The knives of imposter syndrome protruded through my chest, little 'Alicia-From-The-Past' questioning herself why I was doing this and what I got myself into. My mind was foggy and so busy with its chatter - asking questions, answering questions, and making statements:

'REBIRTH time. Going beyond other people's expectations of me. Avoiding limitations. Creating a better life for my family. Letting go of what I was. Knowing at any given moment, I need to trust myself. Divine peace and harmony surround me. I feel compassion and health for all people around me. What if I fail.... Oh, but WHAT IF I FLY?' So much mind-noise!

"LET'S GET STARTED!" A high-pitched voice deep within me fired out. A little hyperactivity sets in. This time with extra energy, I feel myself come back into the present moment, back into my room full of people standing on mini-tramps looking at me for guidance. "LET'S DO THIS"! I now issue lack-of-restraint excitement.

"Let's Do This!" the wonderful warm human beings that make up the crowd echoed back with intensity.

Starting a business is hard! Juggling with little kids is even more challenging. I am only one week from purchasing my new business, and I have already realized people will talk about you, compare you to others, and use you. I am shocked. It is hurtful and unexpected to be viewed only as a service, not as a person anymore. I find myself worrying more than I ever have. My to-do list is more extensive than ever before! I need to remember to respond to all the emails that await me. If I have not posted on my social network immediately, will haters be writing nasties? I find myself in a very anxious state. Will I disappoint someone? Will they hold that against me? Even in a time-sensitive way, I just cannot get to everyone's messages and emails immediately.

WHAT AN EYE-OPENER!

I am a doting Mother of four exceptional children and a wife to a most dedicated, caring & loving human, Mat. I am a daughter, sister, and so much more. I need to be the director of our company, the instructor, the admin, the marketing team, the accountant, and the cleaner, all the while being a mum, a family member, and a loyal, loving, attentive friend.

Can I ask the world kindly for some patience and space? How do I traverse all the chaos? Embrace it? That is all I know.

We are just ordinary people with hectic lives trying to juggle it all.

I have just finished our fully supported by many other local businesses; I Grand Opening of the Boogie Bounce Mackay event yesterday to wake up today with half my family unwell. So much new exposure to our 'Bounce-family classes,' I am forever thankful.

MY FAMILY WILL ALWAYS COME FIRST!

I need to pull off another success without any pushback from myself. Well, this is not a good day; yes, suffered for over two decades with imposter-life-thinking.

IMPOSTER.

I still need to catch up on everything from the event, including my Thank You posts on social media. I appreciate every single one of the small businesses that have supported us, and they all know I would, without any hesitation, do the same for them. I am excited but need help focusing on all I need to do. I am still madly purchasing more signage and tramps, learning new choreography, and putting ourselves through more courses to offer more services.

I wear my heart on my sleeve and know that the most significant learning curve will be that I cannot please everyone. I take everyone's opinions, suggestions, and recommendations on board because I grew up with a stern father, a broken man I always tried to impress. Everything always needed to be better.

I just want to be me. Allow us as a family to run this amazing business so we all can thrive in health and wealth. We would love to retire Mat from his current work, have him work full-time with me in Boogie Bounce, and create the lifestyle we want to live for our family and friends so we can support others and the charities dear to us.

Cross-pollinating like Little Bees supporting each other in small local businesses is the golden key. Making many friends in business, there is plenty of room for everyone to thrive, even in the same industry - this is my biggest wish for people to acknowledge. To share and collaborate and support each other's ventures. I have learned to stay in my lane and stay humble. Let us join together and excel - you're capable - anything is possible with support. Staying in my lane allows me to focus on my strengths and understand, grow, and develop myself. No one must be perfect. Offering myself a more precise direction to increase my productivity in a clear scope. CLARITY - something I have struggled with. My not paying attention all the time, my fidgeting, my lack of restraint, my impatience, and my not following things through stems from my ADHD (attention deficit hyperactivity disorder). I know this but authentically work with it all in my lane.

Previously with my ADHD, I have found it challenging to stick to one thing. Impulsivity and mood swings are all a part of it. I am impulsive. Start many things, jump from one to another: In my career processes, I would blow up one balloon half full, then start another & another, more, all half full. I realized I had all these half-filled balloons I was struggling to keep afloat and yet no full ones. I have been historically impulsive. Other people were getting around with their full balloons, and I had all my half balloons and struggling. Time to let all those half-filled balloons go, watch them fly off into the sky, and pump up my one Bounce Balloon now, on the rebound.

Embracing the chaos.

A little 'me time' I love to read romance novels, a wonderful and dramatic escape; I have always been a fan of chivalry & courting. Actions speak louder than words, marked by honor, acts of love and generosity, graciousness, courtesy, and high-minded consideration are in short supply these days. I love novels from the 1800s, whereby things can be ironic and witty. I love stories with a narrative that may say one thing yet mean another, even psychoanalytical, like my favorite, Pride and Prejudice, by Jane Austen. Chivalry is a dying breed.

The major heartaches in my life? LOTS, so many, I need to list them. They all previously defined me. I have been known to dwell in the past. This has caused me many significant losses in my life. History took control of my life - I sat in self-pity, and yet I realized nobody was saving me. No one is coming. This is an inside job, and I must keep myself.

I have made it out of many situations, too many to recall. My past now does not define me.

My brothers and I grew up together, only each other to lean on. One brother commented that we lived on a different path and traveled a different road to other kids, a route that he felt 95% of the world's kids' upbringing was great. We were the 5% of a Sh*^Ty one.

Self-pity. I sat in that for twenty years. It has interfered with relationships and careers, ended romantic relationships, and caused so much heartbreak and permanent scars. - *no one was coming, Alicia!*

Self-sabotaged yet again. I was packing my whole world up, all the things I loved and owned, sitting in my ex-boyfriend's bedroom with my Mother. Trying to squish into my first car, my Kermit Beetle Green Love Bug, my TV, and everything else important to me, bawling. Everything was so YUK. I had no words. Still so painful to take me back to those memories. A pivotal moment in my life - Save me—time to change.

Other pivotal moments in my life? Our beautiful eldest son being born into this world is a fantastic moment. Our children, 4 including twins, are now my life's true gems and loves. My doting partner Mat loved me from day dot. Has backed me during all that we have endured. 'WE' is our new business; in this family-oriented business, we are ready to thrive from within.

I have always loved the health & beauty industry and wholeheartedly believe health is from the inside out.

I started my hairdressing apprenticeship, worked at a Tea-and-Tidy for many years, and started my Diploma in Beauty, but then life got in the way. My impulsiveness took the reins, and I started all that useless balloon-blowing.

We now embrace the chaos together; through it all, the intention is to arrive at divine peace within this chaos. We can have it all in a tolerant and inclusive way.

The journey begins.

What will I be once Mat and I hit our goals AFTER our transformation? We will be us!

The golden moments lay within the journey, *within*. Inner work and inner thoughts can hijack any situation, inner turmoil of other people's opinions, and me wanting to please everyone and make it all ok. MY INNER VOICE and all that 'imposter-syndrome-ness' that comes and goes. I resonate with Elizabeth Bennet in my favorite book, Pride and Prejudice. Dealing with preconceived opinions, and social expectations, I realize other people's comments have colored my perception of myself and our world. Still, we all possess a shared flaw - prejudices are quickly formed. Recognizing one's faults, or past pain, irrevocably releasing before it is too little, too late.

"I could easily forgive his pride if he had not mortified mine" - Pride and Prejudice, Jane Austen, 1813, chapter 5.

The admission of some flaws, inward work, and transformation, just like Elizabeth and Darcy, where the theme of pride is acknowledged, but prejudices are quickly formed due to emotional reactions and behavior with no clear vision for the future. In the contrast between care of perception and care for internal values, I have explored this only after writing this.

Am I the sum of my past? NO.

I FEEL LIKE I'VE LIVED IN A SHADOW. BOTH MY OWN & OTHERS. YOU ARE YOUR PERSON; NEVER BE PUNISHED FOR OTHER PEOPLE'S ACTIONS.

Realizing my inner nature, my flaws and mistakes do not define us; leave it be. BE your beautiful self NOW.

What has changed me? The loss of my father and my mother-in-law Cheryl. The realization of how short life is. We only have one life - make it happen. In August 2021, my father died suddenly, and in July 2022, we unexpectedly lost Mat's Mother. I had always assumed Cheryl would be here in our lives & my father left us with many unanswered questions. I want to make things happen at a pivotal moment for Mat and me, we are now in our 30s, and all this sudden loss felt cruel. We had not had the chance to grieve adequately. Mat's Mother was in the same ward as my father was, and I thought I was living it all over again as I went up daily to visit her - Deja Vu.

No more self-doubt.

The rare breed.

Mat calls me a Rare Breed. The definition means 'someone unusual in some way.' I am a virtuoso of helping others. I genuinely love helping people; maybe I am a rare species. I find excellent self-reward inside the energy of assisting others. My greatest virtue would be to defy everything that conventional wisdom tells me. ADHD brings many things with it, and as an adult, it is interesting to list the attributes, but what's wrong with that? We all have different characteristics, right? Rebellious, Audacious, Obsessed, Hot-blooded, Hypnotic, and Emotional. I know few are like me; that is what sets me apart; I know this.

'Admirable' I am told I am; people have told me it is damn hard work. "Intense" and "uncommon," I say Thank you!

My pet peeve is that some of life's noises, like mouth noises and chewing, drive me mad. It is a real thing. Misophonia. Causes me solid emotions, and I do react to these trigger sounds. It affects me. I shake; it makes me so uncomfortable. Such strong feelings rise (like I want to hit them in the mouth - of course, I would not, but the surface is there, no doubt, recurrent conditioning from my younger years.

My New Rules of wellness?

In our household, old rules of constant critiquing are over. Now, new rules around health and wellness are formed. We recognize empowerment outside of perfectionism. Nothing is perfect; we are who we are, being a rare breed.

My parents were regimented and scheduled. I am not. I take mental health days with each of our four children on alternate days to spend magical 1:1 time, mummy and child time—a radical thing to do, maybe, with a more profound point of view. LIFE IS CHAOS, but we love this revolutionary hero inside my head. In some ways, we are all imposters at times. You are not alone—no more measuring yourself against other people's measure of success.

I now find myself sneaking up on my thoughts, *sneaking up on myself.* I had constantly looked over my shoulders for so many years; it's this feeling of calling myself out, this life imposter-life-thinking. From the inside out, I have learned a sense of unworthiness and phoniness; even highly motivated people don't believe the credit is due. Anxiety, Perfection, Self-doubt, and Fear of failure slip in if unattended thoughts run riot. I wonder if this is the time I stand in my recognition. (What if I don't deserve this? Anything that comes my way is a mistake) I call myself out on it and recognize it, release the old programming from serious conflict- this is the trauma response. I am not my old self now.

Live. Fail. Ask for help. Love. Assist others. Community and support. Connection.

What is my wellness mindset? Something that sets me apart is to make everyone feel welcome. Time to put all the old thoughts and medication on that backburner and historical depressive states and set up an all-inclusive life. Having a crappy day? Come and Boogie and Bounce with me. I have found my calling, not just a career or a business.

I am my self-testimony, and with all my hardships, I've made mistakes and obstacles, I've learned wisdom that I've gained, and the fragmented pieces of me have come together. I am starting now from where I am; if I can help someone else with my passions and strength, the rest is easy. Initially, turning up is the hardest thing. You're not alone. The beginning of the journey is tough. I am still where you are and ready for the Bounce to return. What is at stake if we don't empower each other? Tapping in and turning on, let that imposter syndrome be called out so a happy life can be established. Tell someone else, "You're good at that," " That smile looks good on you," or " I see your energy." It's so lovely to be able to relate on a direct level.

My life improves daily. How? I'm on a journey too. How do you feel? Like I am on a path of growth, starting over and again, leaving the old me behind, and instilling trust in myself so that others can trust me and feel trustworthy. My relationships also growing daily. Highlight my achievements daily, too—the realization you don't have to be perfect, like all these Instagram posts you see. People thriving and driving flashy cars, applying expensive potions, and buying Bitcoin-funded-millionaire live, I am being my authentic self. This is me leading from my heart. Being me daily, journaling along a positive path with my family, together, with my clients, and with everyone I can help. Now taking my energy worldwide in Authorship and sending my wellness messages across the globe. What do my clients desire the most? To know, even on the worst day, come and bounce it out. Come and sweat, yell, and sing to the music we bounce to; go and gather together and share REALISTIC energy. JUST BE YOU AND FEEL you are not alone. My work and vision create a positive ripple effect of change.

I'd love to connect with you, even for a chat. Reach out to me, and if you're near Mackay, Far North Queensland, Australia, come to my energetic Boogie Bounce class.

There is plenty of work to be done, looking through a lens of honesty and caring. Let's do it together, bounce in another direction blowing up only on a giant balloon.

About the Author

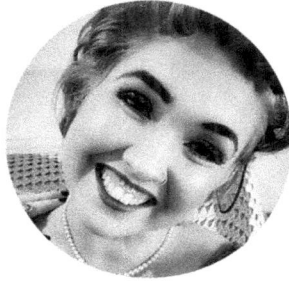

Ally Cashen is a passionate businesswoman, acquiring her certifications as a Personal Trainer, Group Fitness Instructor, and soon-to-be Certified Nutritional Coach in Mackay, far north Queensland, Australia.

Her passion extends beyond her Boogie Bounce Mackay business to Hair, Skin, and Beauty, offering clients the chance to be pampered and advised with body-positive and female empowerment. Her expertise, knowledge, and experience extend to skincare, makeup, and well-being.

Her family is her world. Her husband Mat and four children all enjoy the beautiful Whistsunday outdoors; she volunteers locally and wholeheartedly supports local businesses and enterprises. Ally is affectionately known as 'Our Hype-girl'!

Website: www.gymcatch.com/app/provider/4431
Email: boogiebouncemackay@gmail.com
Facebook: Boogie Bounce Mackay | Facebook

-ᴠᴠᴠ→

Amy Charbonneau

I stood in my bedroom, engulfed by a surge of emotions—hatred and despair instantly consuming me. It felt as though my life would never improve; broken relationships and depression seemed to be an inevitable part of my future. "How did I get here?" I wondered.

I questioned why depression had become a part of my reality. Until that moment, I had never experienced such deep pain and hatred. These unfamiliar feelings overwhelmed me, and the thoughts racing in my mind frightened me. I hated myself for many reasons, despite actually liking who I was. Something inside me was out of alignment, and I couldn't comprehend it.

I had always believed that God created every person with a purpose, endowed with gifts, talents, and passions that the world desperately needed. Yet, as I was ugly-crying on the floor, I began querying this fundamental belief.

"Why me? I can't handle this!" I cried out to God.

"You are not alone," a gentle voice spoke to me.

In that moment of realization, I understood how someone else's trauma had triggered the trauma I had experienced in my own life. Until then, I had never considered that I, too, had trauma. It was just my life—nothing out of the ordinary. But it became evident that I needed help.

Turning to God, I sought His guidance, and His Spirit led me toward profound heart healing.

In the book of John, specifically chapter 16, I discovered that God's Spirit would guide me into all truth. This truth-identity journey began with finding a counselor who shared my beliefs and worked in partnership with God's Spirit. Only through Jesus could I unearth the roots of my pain. I realized an outside perspective plays a vital role in our healing process.

My counselor recommended EMDR therapy (eye movement desensitization and reprocessing), which initially sounded terrifying and unconventional.

"What are they going to do to my brain?" I wondered.

But deep down, I knew it was what I needed.

After my first session, I realized that this rewiring of the brain aligned with what the Message Bible describes in Romans 12:1-3:

"So, here's what I want you to do, God helping you: Take your everyday, ordinary life—your sleeping, eating, going to work, and walking-around life—and place it before God as an offering. Embracing what God does for you is the best thing you can do for him. Don't become so well-adjusted to your culture that you fit into it without thinking. Instead, fix your attention on God. You'll be changed from the inside out. Readily recognize what he wants from you and quickly respond to it. Unlike the culture around you, always dragging you down to its level of immaturity, God brings the best out of you and develops well-formed maturity in you.

I'm speaking to you out of deep gratitude for all God has given me, especially as I have responsibilities concerning you. Living then, as every one of you does, in pure grace, it's essential that you not misinterpret yourselves as people bringing this goodness to God. No, God brings it all to you. The only accurate way to understand ourselves is by what God is and by what he does for us, not by what we are and what we do for him."

Throughout my therapy, I addressed various traumatic events, including divorce, remarriage, a suicidal moment, an abortion, and adoption.

It amazed me that feeling like a new person only took seven

sessions. I realized that this was what it meant to take my thoughts captive, something that had always eluded me in the past (2 Cor. 10:5). I decided to help as many women as possible to find the root of their pain and experience freedom, joy, peace, and love.

Reflecting on my journey, I have overcome struggles with divorce, single parenting, a new husband, and a deepening faith. Yet, despite these victories, depression, fear, and anxiety still lingered in my life. It was a puzzle I couldn't solve, a barrier I couldn't break through until I reached out for help.

I read books about inner healing that spoke to my heart and realized that my true calling was to help women feel amazing. As I read through the powerful stories of transformation and healing, I couldn't help but be overwhelmed with a sense of purpose and a calling that resonated deep within me. The words on the pages spoke to my heart, igniting a fire within my soul. I knew my true calling was to help women find the root of their pain and guide them toward experiencing freedom, joy, peace, and love.

This is who I am! It has been my nature since I was a little girl. I always loved giving makeovers to my family and friends. That passion led to a career in Cosmetology, where I got to help women look and feel amazing! As I grew, my heart for others to know their beauty turned inward. I want others to know they are beautiful from the inside out. I began to lead a transformational women's group.

My vision for impact was born!

I know that my life calling involves helping one more person get off the floor of despair. It can be excruciating to watch those I encounter remain stuck in their vortex of chaotic emotions when there is a way out! When I was stuck, I needed someone to show me, Hope. A friend called me out. She recognized I was not getting anywhere, and even though she did not personally have the tools to help me, she recommended me to someone who had the skills and training to help me move from where I was to where I wanted to be.

If we could sit down or go for a walk, I could tell you all the fantastic stories of how I am a different woman, the more authentic version of me than I had been in decades. Emotional pain debilitated my life. I moved slower, dreamed less, and even worse…believed less.

Joy has returned to my life. Every day I function from an ability to be in the circumstances, good and bad, and return to joy quickly, mentally and emotionally. When frustration, sadness, grief, anger, or any other negative emotions surface, I know how to use them as a meter and handle my heart and mind.

Deep pain and deep healing are emotionally exhausting; achieving freedom takes intentional mindfulness and diligence. I offer patience, grace, and permission to grieve but also stress the importance of commitment and intentionality. Paramount to any profound heart transformation, I talk about Jesus and all He does for us spiritually.

Here are a few stories from women I have helped to see something they could not see.

(Names have been changed to protect identity).

Ruth—"In February 2021, I had a powerful encounter with God that completely liberated me from the heavy bondage I was carrying, and it opened my eyes to the fullness of Jesus. While navigating my newfound life in Christ, Amy played a crucial role in my journey. Her handling of my curiosities, questions, and concerns was beautiful. Even to this day, the memories of her support bring tears to my eyes and an overwhelming sense of gratitude. Amy was there for me when I needed her most. After my encounter, I started experiencing visions and receiving prophetic words from God, but I felt confused and unsure of what was happening. During a retreat a few months later, I stood near a sick friend as others gathered around, laying hands and praying for her. At that moment, I was overwhelmed by a strong sensation in my hands, almost like lightning coursing through me. I didn't know how to handle it and began to panic. Amy looked up, sensing my distress, and gently instructed me to lay my hands on our friend and pray. She reassured me that what I was experiencing was normal and guided me through that powerful moment. Amy has been a gentle shepherd in my life countless times, always showing me the way without judgment or criticism. I honestly don't know where I would be without her. She is a true blessing, not only in my life but in the lives of many others. I thank the Lord every day for placing Amy in my path. Her presence and guidance have made a significant difference, and I am forever grateful."

Beth —Beth approached me because she had endured extensive trauma from her childhood, resulting in deep pain and a sense of distance in her closest relationships. As we embarked on the journey towards joy, she discovered profound healing and courageously took brave steps into her future. It became apparent that her troubled relationship with her adoptive mother was a significant source of her emotional distress. We recognized the need for inner healing through prayerful guidance and open conversations. We scheduled a dedicated 2-hour session to address the painful memories that had created a blockage between her and her mother. During this session, we delved into the depths of her past, working through the wounds and finding pathways to healing.

In her heartfelt words, she said, "You helped me heal from the traumatic experiences of my childhood that had been holding me back. You embraced and loved me as I was, profoundly impacting my healing journey." Witnessing the transformative power of healing and being a compassionate guide is a privilege. This woman's story is a testament to the profound impact of addressing and healing past trauma on one's present and future. I am grateful to have played a part in her journey toward wholeness and restoration.

I embarked on a journey of leading a transformational women's group where women could unite, share their stories, and support one another in their pursuit of healing and wholeness.

Deep pain requires deep healing, and I understand the emotional exhaustion and diligence it takes to achieve true freedom.

I offer my clients patience, grace, and permission to grieve while emphasizing the importance of commitment and intentionality in the healing process. And at the core of it all, I emphasize the role of Jesus and His transformative power in our lives.

To provide a glimpse of the impact of this work, I shared stories from women I have helped along their journeys. Ruth, who experienced a powerful encounter with God, found support and guidance through our interactions. Her memories of my presence brought tears to her eyes and a profound sense of gratitude. Beth, who had endured deep childhood trauma, discovered the healing and the courage to navigate her future with renewed hope.

These stories testify to the transformative power of addressing and healing past traumas, and I feel privileged to play a part in their journeys toward wholeness and restoration.

Nothing is worse than wanting emotional healing for someone more than they want it! I have watched people I love choose not to do this work, and it grieves my heart to see them continue in a hindered life! I pray that they will seek help one day, and I encourage you to do the same.

In my coaching program, I guide women to embrace their true selves, discover their unique gifts, and learn to share their stories with the world. Through one-on-one coaching, short-term goal setting, and inner healing sessions, I provide the support and perspective needed for women to navigate their path toward emotional freedom.

I understand the importance of an outside perspective, someone who could offer a fresh viewpoint and guide others through their darkest moments. Sometimes life feels like we are sitting on a train track, trying to get to the other side, but all we can see are the fast-moving train cars speeding past us. We experience impatience and overwhelm as we wrestle with waiting in the stillness while we want the adventure on the other side! Like a friend in a helicopter overlooking the first to the last cars at a train track, I aimed to be that person who could see beyond the immediate obstacles and encourage others to hold on a little longer.

A learner at heart, I am passionate about continually expanding and applying my knowledge to bring about real change. Knowledge alone is only sufficient with practical application. And above all, my love for people fuels my desire to impact their lives positively. The scripture in Psalm 139 reminds me that each person is fearfully and wonderfully made, created to inspire awe and wonder. You and I are unlike anyone or anything else in all of creation! That is an incredible picture! You have immeasurable value to the world around you.

Though my journey has been painful, it led me to start my own company, focusing on creating a safe and healthy environment for physical healing. Awaken Joy Skincare and Awaken Joy Spice Co were born to provide others with medicinal and therapeutic products and nourishing experiences.

My husband and I were trying to film a clip from him for our Spice Club members, and we could not stop laughing!!! We were on a trip in California, just the two of us (something that had not happened for 16 years). As we walked along this gorgeous river, we decided it was the perfect spot to shoot a few short videos for our business. My husband, a man of quiet countenance, could not stop laughing!!!! You can find the video on our Instagram page (@awaken_joy_spice_co). I hope it makes you smile. But beyond the products and businesses, my greatest joy comes from spending time with my husband, who shares my love for people and food. Our laughter-filled days are a testament to our marriage's vibrancy and shared faith in Jesus.

Awaken Joy Skincare will soon be offering courses or downloadable instructions to help our global readers have access to create their own lovely, non-toxic products that have been tested and approved by thousands of clients. You can find links below to follow us and stay connected.

Spices are a fabulous way to add extra health benefits to your day. For thousands of years, spices were used as medicine (and still are in some regions). Spices were once a form of currency! I giggle, thinking about going to Amazon and saying, "Will you take 5 pounds of basil for that????"

I mean, seriously—how far we are from spice as currency, yet humanity has valued that which serves us best. Spices not only flavor food, but they also help heal your body and brighten your spirits. Here is a fun little Curry blend for you to try at home:

Curry blend:

- 1 tablespoon ground cumin
- 1 tablespoon ground coriander
- 1 tablespoon ground turmeric
- 1 tablespoon ground ginger
- 1 tablespoon ground paprika

- 1/2 teaspoon ground cinnamon
- 1/2 teaspoon cayenne pepper (optional)

Cumin is rich in antioxidants and has anti-inflammatory properties, helping to reduce inflammation and improve digestion.

Coriander is an excellent source of vitamins, minerals, and antioxidants. It may even have antimicrobial properties, aiding digestion, promoting healthy cholesterol levels, and supporting overall heart health.

Turmeric contains a powerful compound called curcumin, which has potent anti-inflammatory and antioxidant properties. It may help reduce chronic inflammation, support joint health, and improve brain health.

Ginger has long been used for its medicinal properties and is known for its ability to soothe digestive discomfort, reduce nausea, and relieve inflammation and muscle soreness.

Paprika is rich in antioxidants, mainly a compound called capsaicin, which may help boost metabolism, promote weight loss, and provide pain relief.

Cinnamon has been linked to various health benefits, including helping to regulate blood sugar levels, reducing inflammation, supporting heart health, and potentially boosting cognitive function.

Cayenne pepper also contains capsaicin, which gives it its spicy heat. Capsaicin has been shown to relieve pain, boost metabolism, aid digestion, and potentially promote heart health.

This blend adds flavor and offers unique health benefits that can enhance overall well-being (something we shoot for at Awaken Joy, LLC).

To the person reading this chapter, I want you to know that you are not alone. I have written these words for you, someone who may feel unheard and misunderstood. I am here, ready to offer an outside perspective to help you navigate your path toward freedom and realize your purpose.

No matter where you are in the world, just a Zoom call away, my NEW RULE OF WELLNESS is to help you discover God's plan for your life, experience His deep love, and receive the healing your heart craves. Together, we can change the world, one heart at a time.

You can find us at the following links:

https://awakenjoyskincare.com
https://awakenjoyspiceco.com/start--for our spice blends
https://awakenjoyspiceco.com/monthly-for our monthly spice club

https://awakenjoyleadership.com/coaching-home
https://www.instagram.com/awaken_joy_spice_co
https://www.instagram.com/awakenjoyskincare
https://www.instagram.com/awakenjoyleadership

About the Author

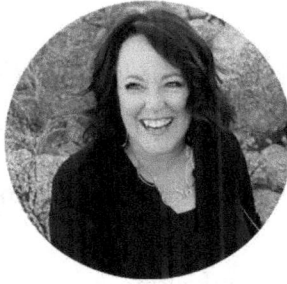

Amy Charbonneau has been working in the Holistic Wellness industry for over 23 years and, as a result of piecing her life puzzle together, is now proudly owning and running Awaken Joy, LLC: Coaching, Spice Co, and Skincare. Amy and her family reside in the USA.

She and her husband are now providing valuable support, culinary expertise, and writing a new cookbook. Amy values diversity and firmly believes every person is made to enhance the earth. She delights in helping people step into their power with permission to thrive.

International Best-selling author: *Art of Connection, a global entrepreneurial endeavor.*

Contributing Author: *The Art of Connection.*

Scars to Star-speaking to those who have been impacted or struggled with Suicide.

Supporting her husband's coming Cookbook: *A Father's Hug from the Kitchen*

> *"Inspiring people to do hard things"*
> - Amy Charbonneau

Digital Home Page: https://mydigitalhomepage.com/amy-charbonneau/

Website: https://awakenjoyskincare.com

Instagram: Amy Charbonneau (@awakenjoyskincare)

-ᴠᴠᴠ→

Michelle Cogley

PART A

The unknown

My two Angels wrap themselves around me and guide me through this stage in life where my old self is gone, just a memory that echoes in my mind, and my new self is still finding her feet and working out how she fits into this world. She isn't fully born yet, but like a Phoenix rising from the ashes, she is still incredibly powerful with a will to survive beyond her comprehension. I talk to Diesel & Lahli daily, listening and watching for the signs that they are beside me, walking this next chapter with me, and I know they are there. My baby boy and tiny little girl give me the strength to forge ahead and continue my path into the unknown. I stare at their photos; my heart is heavy, and I taste the saltiness of my tears streaming down my face; flooded with emotions, I smile, a light-hearted laugh between my soul and I, the irony that we can feel contrasting emotions simultaneously and the reflection of this throughout my life and in the future that awaits me.

In my darkest days, I always knew I would share this with the world. They say "Everything happens for a reason" "Life never gives you more than you have the strength to deal with," but really? Does it? One thing those sayings do is frustrate the hell out of someone who feels broken and alone, the last thing they need to hear is a bloody saying from a Hallmark card.

Did this happen because I'm not afraid to speak out and use my voice? Was there a divine knowing, or am I just trying to make sense of it all?

I know that I AM NOT ALONE in my pain and that my story needs to be heard.

JOURNAL ENTRY: June 2022.

Shining a light on our story forces it out of the shadows; without darkness, our shame, fear, and anger have nowhere to hide. They are stark naked and stripped of their power, and my only responsibility is to speak from my heart. Managing other people's fear and judgment is not my job; those ready to hear I will listen, and my energy is too precious to worry about those who are not.

I walk up the stairs, confident and proud, ready to speak to the hearts of everyone in the audience. I am so grateful for the experience, and I never considered my neurological symptoms might be triggered tonight. The overstimulation of the bright lights and the noise had sent my body into unseen mayhem thank goodness I could use the podium to hold myself up. I am deeply honored to be a guest speaker on Dr. Malhotra's National tour, and as I cast my eyes out into the crowd, I see them waiting with open hearts. They are ready; I take a deep breath and share my story.

I stand here today as the collateral damage of a broken system.

Today I am a voice to honor those who are no longer with us, for those of us that are too unwell to get out of bed each day, and for those still too afraid to speak out.

My story is like so many others. It's a story full of pain, frustration, heartbreak, and grief, but It's also a story of courage, resilience, and hope.

In October 2021, I got my first Pfizer vaccine. Within 5 minutes, my heart started racing, and I felt nauseous. The nurse looked at me and asked if I was ok? As she started walking towards me and I stood to meet her, my body felt weak, and I collapsed. I was helped onto a chair and given an oxygen mask, and the nurses tried to tell me, 'This is just anxiety.' I knew this was NOT anxiety. After being monitored for more than 30 minutes, my symptoms were not reduced, It was clear that this was not anxiety but also that they had no intention of investigating further, so I took myself home. As I walked in the front door, I felt a sudden rush come over me; I bolted to the sink and vomited repeatedly for the next 10 minutes.

Over the next three weeks, I experienced mild symptoms, sharp pains in my chest, and some shortness of breath while the symptoms were out of character at this stage, they were mild and, in my mind, not significant enough for me to take myself to the doctors or hospitals.

At that stage of the pandemic, the mandates specified that a 2nd vaccine must be given 3 weeks later, I had held out until the very last moment in hopes that I wouldn't have to get it but it was fast approaching the cut-off date for when Vets would no longer allow the unvaccinated to go in with their animals. I could deal with being excluded from society but my animals are my family, my everything, and as their mother not being by their side in their Time of need was a risk I was unwilling to take, so 3 weeks on, I went and had my second Pfizer vaccine, a decision that would change the trajectory of my life.

After my first reaction, I was concerned about what could happen. My mum came with me and stood by my side, offering me the comfort I needed the way only a mother can. My dad's lineage has a strong history of heart-related issues, which was at the forefront of my mind. I told the nurse the symptoms I had experienced over the previous 3 weeks and asked if I could proceed. In a calm voice, she said, "Well, you haven't been hospitalized, so you still need to have the second vaccination. Even if you get peri or myocarditis, you will get over it quickly, and you will be fine".

It was at that moment I wish I had listened to my intuition, the voice inside of me that told me this wasn't right for me, but instead, I chose to close my eyes, cross my fingers, and hoped that'd be ok.

Throughout the day, I started getting random sharp pains and a bit of tightness in my chest, so that night, I took myself to bed early in hopes that it would resolve itself by morning. At 4 am the next day, everything changed!

I woke up suddenly and felt like I had been hit by a truck. My heart was racing, my skin was clammy, my body was shaking, and I was in agony. My heart felt like it was about to beat out of my chest, and as I struggled for air, it felt like I had a vice wrapped around my ribcage, squeezing me, and like someone was sitting on top of me smothering my mouth to try and stop me from breathing.

I was drenched in fear, shame, and denial as I thought, "Please don't let this be real." As the morning continued, my symptoms got worse. My heart rate sat at a constant 160-170 bpm just sitting on the couch. I had sharp pains in my chest, neck, back, and arms, so I called an ambulance.

As I lay in the emergency alone, covered in electrodes all over my chest, the doctor told me they had ruled out a heart attack. She was rushing, and it appeared she had no time for questions; she was already halfway out of the room when she gave me the diagnosis:

"You have Pericarditis."

I said back to her, "Can you please stop? What does this mean? How long will I be affected, and what do I do from here?" Her response... 'We just need to get you out of here.'

That first trip to the emergency left me speechless. It was horrible and completely dismissive.

Dosed up on morphine, with no way of getting home, I didn't know exactly where I was, and they were rushing me out the door into the pouring rain. I knew the hospital, but I had never been there before; I had lost my bearings and couldn't find where to go. My mum, my savior found her way to me, and as I stepped into the dry warmth of her car, I sat stunned in shock as the tears welled in my eyes, I looked at her, and I saw the pain in hers while we drove back home in disbelief.

Back in the comfort of my home, Diesel lay beside me as my cats gathered around.

Surrounded by a vortex of love, I did my best to surrender to the pain. As I tried to sleep that night, I clutched my phone, ready to call for help. I slept sitting up because the pressure on my chest was too great to lie down; little did I know this was how I would sleep for many months to come. In the following days, the pain was excruciating. I couldn't stand long enough to make a cup of tea without my body giving way, I could not talk and breathe without gasping for air, and the sharp shooting pains wouldn't stop. Three days later, I was back in an emergency after collapsing at the doctor's while waiting in line.

As the other patients tried to help me up, they realized there was nowhere to help me because all the chairs had been cordoned off, and the staff was behind big screens, so they couldn't see what had happened. When the medical team arrived and helped me into a wheelchair, I tried to get the words out, "I have pericarditis from the vaccine." However, because I was struggling to speak and still gasping for air through the mandated mask, they talked over the top of me and interrupted me several times, saying, "You just have anxiety." It was again confirmed in an emergency that I had pericarditis from the vaccine, which was NOT anxiety.

I sat in wonder, why was this assumption of 'Anxiety' being thrown around so loosely? I overheard the nurses debriefing the doctor behind the curtain. 'Another vaccine reaction in bed 14, her second time here in 3 days'. After being sent home with drugs for my pericarditis and to help with my pain, I returned to my GP with the discharge papers in hand the next day. Still in significant pain and unable to speak correctly because of the pressure on my chest, I asked if I could have the referrals for an echocardiogram and cardiologist as requested by the emergency doctor. My GP looked at me and said:

"No, I don't think you need it; you will get over it within a week"

I sat there in shock.

How could she not see how bad I was?

I was struggling to breathe; I couldn't stand up, I could barely talk, I had the feeling of knives constantly stabbing me, and my chest felt like it was burning from the inside out. Her response just didn't make sense. We sat there in a weird stare, looking at each other over the top of our masks I held her stare, refusing to be intimidated by her scowl "How much worse do I have to get for you to take me seriously?"

As a vaccine injured, we are not just faced with the challenge of getting our health back; we are also fighting a system to get recognized medically and find someone to help us get answers. On top of that, we are faced with the constant bias of society and, for many, the dismissiveness from their own family and friends.

The stories laced with fear that ran through my mind consumed me. The charged and intense political emotions seemed to have people disconnecting from their humanity and compassion.

In a society so fuelled with opinions, pro-vax, anti-vax, doing whatever you could hold your life together vax, where had our sense of community and connection gone?

Life was a whirlwind of constant doctors and specialist appointments with few answers.

I have had countless tests, and we have tried multiple treatments, but besides a large amount of weight gain and enormous stress on other bodily systems, my body wasn't responding, and the only thing that seemed to be helping was time.

Being someone who has always valued alternative medicine and never entirely understood why it's so difficult for people to use the benefits of both worlds, I longed to be able to support my healing journey with other treatments. Still, the elephant in the room is that no money is coming in when your livelihood has been taken away from you and your most outstanding achievement for the day is standing long enough to cook dinner. People can suggest all the best treatments in the world, but there is no access.

Life as I knew it was gone.

I had gone from being a successful, independent, and driven entrepreneur to losing everything, and it would be a year before I was even strong enough to I volunteer at the local soup kitchen for a few hours to put food on my table.

The first 3-6 months were the most intense and lonely. Every day, I woke up in fear that I wouldn't see the day's end. Part of the reality of severe illness for a person living alone is that a confrontation occurs within your soul, day in and day out. A never-ending cycle and negotiation with your mind in the deafening silence with many emotions all fighting to be the loudest.

JOURNAL ENTRY: February 2022.

I witness you, and you are brave. The wind is here today to help you release the stagnant muck in your soul. I know it doesn't feel good, but there is a lot of old identity to purge. There is no easy way to release it, but you have the strength to go through it. It's in accepting that right now, your physical and cognitive abilities are not what they once were, and with that comes a level of managing your mind that you have not previously had access to. Walk with Diesel in the wind, hold him, meditate and cuddle the cats, nurture your soul today with mother nature, and bathe in your connection.

The road to inclusivity is still being determined. What is it about humans that we become so attached to our opinions, we forget that on the other side of the 'numbers' are people.

Throughout this journey, I have seen many shifts in society, and although it's much slower than necessary, the conversation is changing, which brings hope. Where people once averted eye contact and fidgeted awkwardly at the mere mention of the V word, now more people keep eye contact and lean in to understand and feed their curiosity.

What I can't make sense of is why medically, these cases are not being overseen as a whole. I have been hand-balled from doctor to doctor, told that they have no idea what to do with me.

These cases are complex and frustrating. What started as 1 thing has now snowballed into a myriad of other conditions. "Follow the science," they say; well, WE ARE THE SCIENCE, and not once have we been followed. Years of data are gone, lost opportunities, and no one is Accountable.

JOURNAL ENTRY: December 2021.

My boy Diesel by my side I don't think I could get through this without him. We need love to heal, and without my kids (animals), my mum, and my dad, would I still be standing? Mum and Dad have been thrust into a world where they once again care for and support their daughter, just like when I was a little girl. The impact on them isn't fair. We didn't sign up for this.

Where is everyone? I long for the company of a friend to come and sit with me, watch a movie with me, let me know they care enough to come over, and just simply be with me.

They appreciate many comfort messages, but besides Mum and Dad, it's been weeks, and I haven't seen a soul. We live in a world of so much communication and little human connection. Is this how I've supported people in the past? Have I not realized when a friend needed me? We've all done it, haven't we? Nothing more than a text message when what they needed was physical contact.

Each day I battle a war inside my chest, a pain I have learned to live with. I seek refuge daily through nervous system regulation, but my neurological symptoms persist even in my soul's calmest moments. I can be amid meditation in divine bliss when my body fires off a rapid machine gun of stabbing pains and jolting fireworks. The unseen turmoil bubbling beneath the surface is the daily challenges of extreme fatigue, dizziness, scattered thinking, and cognitive difficulties with my learning, memory, and problem-solving.

There's no sugar-coating it; you can practice all the self-help tools in the world, but sometimes life can be crappy. Back then, I thought I knew pain, but little did I know what was to come and the bomb that was about to go off...

About the Author

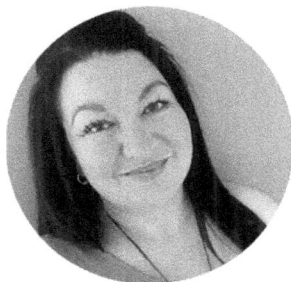

Michelle Cogley has been a Canine Behaviourist for over 16 years and had run her own successful business for over a decade before becoming one of the vaccine injured. With a background in Dog Training and Behaviour, Veterinary Nursing, and Animal Rehabilitation, she has also studied Human Behaviour and Personal Development, Neuro-linguistic programming, Timeline Therapy, and Hypnosis.

Michelle has been a sought-after and respected educator, running workshops, seminars, educational programs, fundraisers, and teaching college students within the animal industry. A career inspired by her boy Diesel, they lived an active lifestyle together and devoted their lives to helping, inspiring, and teaching others about the human/animal bond.

Website: www.animalescapades.com.au
Email: michelle@animalescapades.com.au
Instagram: @animal_escapades_k9

-WW→

Michelle Cogley

PART B

Trust

March 5th 2022, the day I died a million deaths. Life stopped, and every version of me was gone forever. My worst nightmare was here banging down the door. The darkness had arrived and wrapped itself around every breath that I took. I was a fool if I thought I knew pain before this moment.

I lay on the floor beside him, knowing this was the last time we would ever breathe the same air together, the last time I would feel the warmth of his breath against my cheek, the last time he would nuzzle into me, and I would cradle his body as his protector, his soul mate, his Mum.

My boy, I am hollow, I am empty, my soul has left, and I am simply just a body attached to a breathing machine pumping oxygen. Everything is dark, I no longer hear the world; I lay on

the kitchen floor screaming, howling, smashing my fist repeatedly until my body goes limp. The black void engulfs me, and the deep pain in my soul wraps itself around every cell in my body until nothing is left. Michelle died that day, flicking the life switch to autopilot, and now her only purpose was survival.

JOURNAL ENTRY: March 2022.

Diesel, for 17 years, you were my reason for living. I don't know how to do life without you, I don't know who I am without you. You were the one that gave me purpose and direction, and you shaped the person I am today; it's always been me and you, the inspiration for my career every step of the way; we are a team. I don't want to open my eyes every day I wake up. I'm too scared to roll over and see you are no longer there, lying next to me. What do I do now? How the hell do I get through this?

... One hour at a time.

For months to come, when I awoke, I felt the monster, a beast dwelling in the pit of my stomach. I know him well; we have been connected since I was a little girl. He knows my thoughts and feeds off of my soul. He is the part of me that the world doesn't see; he is elusive and quick..... His name is bipolar.

When the monster grabs hold, the world only exists in shades of black and grey, and I had spent many of my younger years vilifying the grey, constantly searching for the colour. In those days, weeks, and months, I would do anything to feel the life-force energy of red, green, and purple. Still, the darkness was so intense, and all the things I would usually do to help myself were out of reach because of this vaccine injury. They were simply silhouetted on a movie screen where one of the main characters was gone, and the one left standing could barely breathe.

Grief is such a mysterious beast, a paralysis of the mind, body and soul overridden only by self-preservation, the pause becomes a freeze, and we are faced with only one choice, keep going or tap out. Faced with the reality that tapping out was not an option, I couldn't do that to my Mum, Dad and my cats, but I had no idea how to keep going. It didn't get easier, I just got better at pretending.

I've learnt over many years some people don't understand mental illness yet are all too willing to give their opinion and dismiss it as someone being depressed or anxious who doesn't know how to get over it or needs to harden up. Depression and anxiety are normal emotions every human feels, but that is not what mental illness is. The day I stopped seeing him as a 'monster' and started to see him as my superpower was the day I reclaimed my worth; thank goodness my younger self embraced that insight because another layer of shame at this time in my life could have been the straw that broke the camels back. I told him I would love him and keep him safe no matter what. There is nothing to be 'Fixed' there is no 'One session, and you'll be cured'. The beast, the monster, is a part of me, and he is beautiful. He helps me to connect more deeply with life; he helps me to see things from multiple perspectives at once. He allows me more self-awareness and encourages me to reflect deeper than any personal development mentor ever could. We live together, we are a team, and our relationship has no room for shame or demonising.

JOURNAL ENTRY: July 2022.

Grief isn't something that happens to you, it becomes you, and now the question is, who are you inside of the grief? The Michelle that existed before now that I was so attached to is gone, and the only way forward is acceptance and finding the strength each day to show up. Some days showing up is nothing more than opening the curtains and having a shower; other days, it's going for a walk for as long as your body allows. Be gentle with yourself, let what you feel pass through you and make grounding yourself daily your number one priority.

Rock bottom doesn't always come with one big punch to the face where suddenly you wake up and declare to the world that enough is enough, and from this day forth, you will swear to 'do better' to 'be better'. I'm sure that's how it is for some people, but for others, rock bottom looks like continuous rolling waves smashing you over and over again until you are beached on the rocks with nowhere else to turn.

With Diesel gone and my health hanging in the balance, the battlefields of my birth father's dementia were getting worse by the day. Dementia is ruthless and has no time for grief or illness, and as Dad's emotional support and the one who oversaw his care, my broken soul had to find a way to show up. There is something that happens to you when you are supporting a loved one with dementia, a sense of urgency that plays on repeat in the back of your mind that you're not doing quickly enough because every day that passes is another day the person you once knew fades into the abyss. Compartmentalising my dad's care was the only way I could stave off the undeniable fear and pain of watching my father fade away. A flamboyant man so full of character and life, he was as tough as they come and lived a thousand lifetimes in one, and now a true entertainer had said 'catch ya later' for the very last time.

Another layer of my identity was gone; nothing felt real. It was as if my autopilot had been turned up to turbo speed, and the self-destruct button dangled in the breeze, just willing me to engage. I had to let myself flatline emotionally and spiritually and go deeper into my consciousness. I needed to surrender to all that was and trust the flicker of light within my soul to come and jump-start my heart again.

Regaining our strength and reclaiming our worth takes more than just sitting in a cave and zenning-out with Buddha. We need conscious awareness of where our focus is going, where we are allowing our energy to seep, and what conversations we are flooding our minds with.

I knew that if I was going to give my body and mind a fighting chance of overcoming the last 10 months, I needed to take the check and eliminate anything from my life that wasn't helping me on the road to recovery. How did I want to spend the rest of my days here on Earth? I knew what I didn't like; I didn't want to be angry and bitter at the world; I didn't want to live out my days in judgement with a concrete wall around my heart, never accessing my compassion and love for life again, I didn't want to spend my future dragging around my baggage from the past, and the only one that could make sure that didn't happen was me.

JOURNAL ENTRY: December 2022.

We don't get to own our pain without owning our part it always starts from within. Healing isn't about becoming our best self it's about learning to love and accept our worst self deeply. A layer of me has been laying dormant, and now it's exposed, naked and raw — business, career, health, finances, Diesel, Dad. I feel stripped bare, but I'm still standing, and my job now is to gather up pieces and work out which ones I want to keep and which I want to create. My power lies in understanding myself well enough to know when to move. I am proud to have honoured my timeline and not anybody else's. I will continue honouring the feelings and be gentle with myself as I release the grip on my past.

Each blow to my heart, both physically and metaphorically, set my recovery back.

My relationship with time has always been questionable, but now time was nothing more than an illusion, and the only thing that resets my clock was my daily walks in nature. Some days my walks consisted of going from the car to the park bench so I could bask in the reality of life beyond the four walls of my house, but mostly I escaped into the forest and took my time immersing myself in the tree's calling, upon their wisdom.

Mothers' intuition is a powerful thing. The lump in your throat and the drop in your stomach tell you something isn't right. As I looked into my little girl's eyes and she meowed back at me, something about her meow didn't sit right. When I got her to the vet, she was fading fast, and fear riddled my body again.

'No, this can't be right, surely she will be fine, yesterday she was just bouncing around and happy'. As I heard the words come out of the vet's mouth, the room went blurry, my blood drained instantaneously, and panic set in. 'Lahli has acute kidney failure, stage 4.'

All my pain came rushing back as I felt another sledgehammer to the heart. I pleaded to myself, 'She will be ok, I just need to nurture her through the next few days and adjust her diet, and we will get through this'. I had nurtured Diesel through kidney disease for 2 years before he passed, and he thrived in life until the very end, so I knew all the things I needed to do. It was up to me to fix this. Two days later, with my girl snuggled into my chest, I waited for Diesel to arrive, then my tiny little warrior took her last breath, and in one foul-swoop, she was gone.

JOURNAL ENTRY: April 2023.

What the fuck just happened? Lahli, where have you gone? This grief is so different to the others. None of them have been the same. I'm in shock; how is this even real? You were my angel, my sweet, sensitive soul; we were so connected and in tune. How you stared at me adoringly with those beautiful eyes made me feel so important. You weren't even 24 hours old when I became your mother and hand-reared you; now, 13 years later, you're gone. That wasn't the agreement.

One of the certainties of life is that nothing ever stays the same. Neither good nor bad experiences are permanent, and sometimes knowing this can bring comfort, but right now was not that time. Our emotions are interesting. As humans, we can get so caught up in pedestaling some and vilifying others, but if we were not meant to experience the full spectrum of emotions, they wouldn't exist. We must remember that the other part of the equation is timing.

Frustration, elation, anger, and joy are just as valid as the last. It's the human condition; there is no bypassing it. Our job is to make peace with our emotions whilst remaining responsible for our behaviour. We can allow ourselves to be the full expression of who we are with all our insecurities and quirks and still stand tall.

There have been a lot of emotions I've needed to sit with. The path has been rocky, but we all have challenges; the context might differ, but the code is the same. Our awareness comes when we listen to the conversations in our minds and notice how we're showing up. Just imagine rocking up to the local barista each day expecting them to smile and be warm and welcoming when every day you show up as an arsehole; at some point, their smile will wane. To be surrounded by kindness and compassion, I must also be kind and compassionate. The entanglement of emotions exists on a spectrum. They are not binary; we can feel multiple emotions at once and still find the courage to move forward with grace to find peace in a world full of chaos.

Falling apart bought with it many layers of fear; the illusion of control had been swept away and I needed to find my way back home. Do I still trust myself? Do I still believe in myself?

The answer was often no, but I knew myself enough to know that my will to survive was strong, so the question became: Do I have what it takes to recreate myself?

The answer was a resounding Yes.

'It's not good or bad, it's just different', the words echo in my head. Diesel was blind for most of his life, and when people would approach us with sadness and pity, I quickly protected our energy field and said to them, "Yes, he is blind, but it's not good or bad it's just different; we get to do life differently, and it's up to us to not make that mean anything and still go out and enjoy the richness of life" Now I was faced with the reality that this was no different and how beautiful that one of the best lessons Diesel ever taught me would become the encouragement I needed to move forward on those days when I became frustrated by my physical and mental limitations or the grief overwhelms me.

The process of recreation starts with our hearts and not with our heads. There is an untamed life force inside each of us, a living, breathing part that whispers gently and calls us towards new possibilities. Your life is yours, and it doesn't belong to anyone else; other people's fears and limitations belong to them don't let your insecurities be the reason you don't explore.

Creation is infinite, but this one precious life in this body you are currently in is not.

Did all this happen to me for a reason? Yes and No. I believe that life happens, and it's normal for us to try and find reason within it, but ultimately it's about what we take from it and do with it that makes the difference. We may have chosen a different path to stay trapped in their circumstances, but I knew that I was always going to do something with it. Strength and courage are not handed out to some of us and not others. They are within every being, both human and animal alike. They are nomadic and can be elusive, but they are ready and waiting, and in your stillness, if you listen carefully, you will hear them whisper, 'Trust me, I won't let you fall'.

About the Author

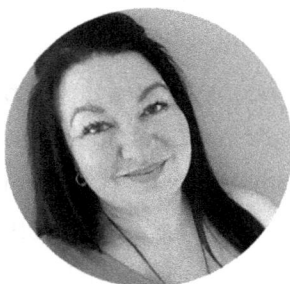

Michelle Cogley is an inspirational keynote speaker and international best-selling author who moves her audience through courage and vulnerability. Renowned for 'keeping it real,' she is a real-life example of how you can ignite your inner strength in the face of controversy and unapologetically reclaim your worth with confidence and compassion.

With a background in animal and human behaviour, Michelle has a unique understanding and a refreshing and raw approach. She is passionate about empowering people to release the layers of shame and fear that come with being human and helping them see their greatness so they can proudly own and live a life they love. To book Michelle for speaking engagements and events, including workshops, fundraisers, seminars, and educational programs, you can contact her on:

Email: mishcogley@icloud.com
Instagram: @mish_cogley
Facebook: https://www.facebook.com/michelle.cogley

-◆-

Merman Andrew Corter

Shello!

I'm Merman Andrew. I love all things water, and this part of my
life is called PEACE. Something that once scared me now calms
me, and submerging in the water is the most peaceful time.
Nothing feels as good as being underwater, at home, igniting my
inner child where everything is novel, beautiful, and filled with
awe, now living out all my forgotten childhood dreams. I love
my pod and all I have created in this magical Mer-World, and
having friends that will dive into your journey is the key. There
are so many reasons to Shell-abrate, being a Merman. You may
wonder how I separate my make-believe world from the real
world—made up. Maybe it isn't? If you look deep into the
waters, you may glimpse a Merman.

My Mer-mazing journey has been a crazy one. It is very different
now from my life which seemed like an eternity ago. Coming
from a corporate job, I was magically transported from its

amalgamated mundanity and disengagement from everyday life into an aquatic world where I would realize I 'shell' never WORK a day in my life again. Filming, performances, brand ambassador work, tank appearances, open-water photoshoots, booked engagements, podcasts, and other interviews, working as a Merman reaches far beyond any life I could have dreamed up. Having a Merman around, everything looks better!

At a corporate function years back, a colleague and I had been in charge of organizing and executing for the company we worked for and had booked a Mermaid that ultimately never showed up. I had a performing arts background and had grown up around a lake where as a young boy, Mom said one day, "Throw him in; he will figure it out" - sink or swim; after the fear left me, I was a water baby. Our sentiment for the no-show-mermaid was,' The show must go on; our function must go on.'

"We have a tail; let's throw it on," I said. Then, hmm, how am I going to do this thought flashed through my head, yet without any hesitation, I donned the tail and did a remarkable job; that day transformed my life.

Living the Merman life takes more than a magic spell to make everything happen.

Swim, dive, endurance training, getting comfortable with the Mono-fin practicing swimming with it, then getting comfortable with being underwater. Diving many feet into the warm, crystal clear ocean waters of Florida, I pick up a 40-pound boulder at the bottom of the ocean floor, similar to how professional surfers train, running with it full speed underwater for a minute, filling my lung capacity, and the depth prepares my body for the pressure. After the drills, I then hold the rock above my head victoriously. Something I feel sets me apart from others; living naturally as possible. I ensure I am eco-conscious and live my entire life that way. I don't go to typical gyms; the water is my gym— rock running, underwater squats, and rock throws. I've learned any gym equipment has an aquatic alternative, and a simple 40-50lb heavy enough rock will keep me on the ocean floor. As a Merman, I share tanks with sharks and fish and often get face slapped by their tails. No day is the same, and nothing is ever a lazy swim. I am not just a brand ambassador, influencer, athlete, or actor. Constantly looking for aquatic-themed jobs and events, new opportunities, and the magic of life becomes me; who knows what's around the corner?

I have O-fish-ally become ME!

Numerous things are essential: safety, professionalism, environmental conservation, inclusion, and activism. My pet peeve is when people do not make this career safe; some do not have the training nor the insurance, and it does scare me that Mermaiding as a profession may be pulled out of an industry due to accidental circumstances. It is, however, a $240 million industry in the USA (2023 market size report USA).

I have my diving PADI certifications for Scuba, Free divers certificate, and a calm heart rate, so I can be more natural in shows and underwater and acclimated to saltwater. PADI course for Mermaids is also essential for knowledge and development of water skills, self-expression aquatic skills, problem management, and confined spaces training. Those tails are cumbersome and 10-foot-long!

At events and photo shoots, I laze on rocks and captivate those watching. In the tank, what do I do? Could you create an ambiance and appeal? As an Aquarium performer, I get into character and create a mental story. I smile a lot, do tricks, wave, blow bubble-kisses, and bubble-rings, swim gracefully, act 'inquisitively' towards my onlookers, interact with them, and follow them as they move past the tank, and when in doubt, POSE!

My work has led me toward marine conservation, supporting Gay-Pride, Reef conservation, and saving our world's reef systems.

GOAL: Diving in The Great BARRIER REEF, Australia.

My many favorite activities as a child always involved water. Growing up on a lake, fishing was a popular pastime, "Put them back," I would yell when we caught a fish.

Suppose I had all the time and money, I'd do more volunteer events for children's hospitals so that the children could see a Merman and have their dreams come true. Kids have grown up watching Mermaid shows and movies– the magic is there with them right when they make a wish; I'd love to continue to spread magic and joy, even if it's just for a moment.

I'd like to see my life story be more of a guardian of the waters! Teaching people about trash dumping in our waterways and springs and getting the knowledge in the community that each piece makes a difference. If one person sees an amount of discarded trash and collects it, an animal won't eat it; the fish won't eat it or get caught in it; a tiny bit of chance to pick up that one piece– just wow! A recent volunteering group collected 40-50lb trash in one body of water - how is that possible? Poor marine life!

I was on the swim team in high school with a supportive family. I haven't been through any significant crises or heartbreaks, which I am thankful for. After winning a lottery draw application to study Performing Arts in Utah, I left my family and state. My love of dance, theater, and dramatic performances has been the building blocks for my amazing life. My work with Disney had me falling back in love with being in front of people and up on stage. My work with some Alcohol brands found me the skills for brand ambassadorship contracts and appearances. It escalated quickly, and I realized I had 33 booked events as a

Merman in Florida, USA. I'm so glad that Mermaid didn't show up that day; the trajectory of my life may have been very different. I connected with the Merman spirit the second I put on that tail and bawled. Some other Mermaids I have spoken to either do or don't; it's an instant thing. Some are 'acting as a job,' others, like me, BECOME. This highlighted the notion that doing cos could change your life if you think about it. This is your reminder to stop procrastinating and change your life!

My journey inside my Merman world is also a sea-riously crazy one!

Early in my career, the first event I worked with, 'Mermaids-and-Marguaritas Festival,' was a land event where I modeled Mer-wear. I had Merman assets and the Mermaid brand Metailor–swimmable Mermaid Tails (I was unaware of the popularity at the time.) "You're wearing leggings and a brand," a voice bellowed at me. I hadn't realized the brand's famous owners and his Mer-wear, oopsy - blush - What The Fin?!

This year, I was called on an emergency booking from Canada, 'Mermaids-Make-Waves, 'at the Aquaterium, Ontario, Canada—my first large Aquarium event, as I am now in love with Aquarium gigs and Large-Tank events.

I loved interacting with the fish, a Mer-person gets in the tank, and the fish are happy and acting natural, and when anything or anyone else gets in the tank, the fish scatter.

I get carried everywhere - up and down stairs - in a cart by Mer-handlers or thrown over their shoulders. I get myself ready and Mer-dressed away from everyone to avoid ruining the magic - no one wants to see me getting dressed from Human to Merman.

The Monofin I step into is like a pair of shoes; the tail skin is difficult and unattractive to put on, but it isn't petty! It's all about embracing the discomfort. The saltwater in the eyes, and the 'do anything to get that perfect shot' mentality. My favorite photographic shoot (my headshot here) was the perfect day, ending not so perfect after the 'perfect' photo; I slid ungracefully off the large rocks, fell between them, and broke my arm. Not for-mentioning as I author this chapter, I had just as ungracefully fallen out of the tree and fractured my Ulna/Radius, and my right forearm is in a cast, BUT, the show must go on. I am figuring out how best to execute my gigs and bookings so I can safely work them all. First up this coming week– a Dunk Tank appearance (Yes, confined spaces). If in doubt, stay in the water; if it feels awkward, it will be amazing!

My family enquires about my job. They are happy that I can pay my bills and thrive. I know they still wonder, 'What else am I going to do' (AKA traditional job!).

I have spent five years building my Mer-brand, getting my name out there, and conservation awareness. Kickbacks? Yes, please.

It's complicated; just because I'm not wearing clamshells as Mermaids do, there are fewer jobs for men, and always elements of social injustice and a lack of inclusion in any professional fields. Initially, I had an identity crisis: Tridents, long hair, beard, large muscles - all weren't me. I purchased a Trident and tried it, but it felt strange; I needed both hands to swim and be flamboyant and super bubbly. THAT Merman image and persona of uber-tough isn't me. I'm' goofy,' 'quirky' - I blew up that image to be authentically me in my Mer-skin. I now strive to be more myself every time, not average but natural, and I learn something every day. Recently I surprised myself; I just happened to exhale in the tank differently and blew bubble rings onto and up the glass; the effect was mes-Mer-rising - I DEVELOPED MY NEW SKILL. Bringing something new to my performances, new tricks. I try to improve each day rather than 'just do a show'; I enjoy it all, maybe a little too much!

What makes this job my career? The creatures and my connection to the water.

I belong.

Sitting on the edge of a tank, I saw the fish come up to the surface to take a look, "Hi there! Oh, you have a tail; come on in"! I hear them say. On other days having not squished me into my tail skin, the fish and creatures come to look, and I can see them frown and swim away. I'm in the tank with sharks; they come to say hello, as all the creatures do. They are all very friendly and welcoming to me; I feel acceptance, they think I belong too, and we are all harmoniously doing our thing.

From inside the tank, everything looks like a blob. DO NOT TAP ON THE GLASS. It's total Bull-Shark! It's confusing and hard to isolate where the noises are coming from; the fish also share my sentiments and person-plant-or inanimate object; either way, I will wave!

In the open water in the ocean, I am still akin to the environment and its creatures, although I find the aquamarine life is a little crazier out there. So many experiences: A sturgeon slapped me in the face; an open water dive had me 'high-fiving' much inquisitive fish, free-diving in a cave, I saw giant eyeballs staring at me - an alligator - and another time, blowing bubbles and bubble kissing what I thought was a cameraman and turned out to be the tail of a giant shark. As I never wear goggles, my vision is blurred, and I've trained my eyes not to sting too much in the salty water. I've learned the art of staying alert, not to jolt-in-surprise to anything, not being fearful, and many 'backing away slowly and calmly' maneuvers.

Yes, we have "Mermaid emergencies." I often get calls to fill in where a Mermaid has fallen ill, contracted a virus, and is out for a week, in a car accident, or other events. My highly scheduled life, including a weekend off now and then, can fall into disarray promptly.

"We need a Mer-person quickly; we need you all weekend!"

You only know what lies beneath the water's surface once you look; remember this when you are in the ocean or a deep pool. Some swimmers were above me, masks on, and then looking down at the ocean floor, and seeing me and my magnificent tail shock them, I swam around and out of sight, and I could see them frantically looking around. I can only imagine the conversations that would be had once back on the beach. Another time at the beach, it got busy with lots of people in the shallows, and it was my first time trying to wrangle my Monofin and tail skin in the sandy environment. It wasn't pretty; I did my best and rolled into the water and swam out. I bobbed and waved about, weaving around people's feet, and flicked a person with my tail, "Hi, I'm so sorry!" I blurted out with just as much surprise as the man, and swam away, doing the 'Merman-launch-into-the-water-flick-of-the-tail' move with no further context. Guarantee he has told his mates on the trip to Florida, " I saw a merman!!"

I'm a fan of fiction and inspirational books, breathing method books, but nothing as passionate stands out as the movies, shows, and Netflix. I, too, have been featured! What has inspired me the most is Mako Mermaids, filmed in Australia, the H20 show, Splash, and the like. The turning point for me was that 'My-Trident-turning-point-of-identity—the exact replica of the show. I was never an underachiever, but I felt it at that exact point. I needed to amp it up - addressing my swim styles and certain techniques. The CGI on those shows had me saying, "I can't do that!!" Water dragons have also impacted my life in more mystical and magical aspects– I love the water dragon story. Books are full of magic, movies are full of charm, and our lives can be full of magic, too, if we choose.

My New Rule for Wellness; Wherever you are and whatever you are doing, be ready.

Be ready to act immediately.

Say YES to that moment that may change your life, that offer or substitution, a chance (no matter how left-of-center it may sound). Be ready to pose, be prepared to smile, and be willing to make another being's life happy too.

Social media has become a passion of mine, an ever-evolving beast of its own. Like the world of 'Mermaiding,' the chance and opportunity to share my mystical and magical days and work, I reach millions of people in one click. This has been very powerful in expanding my business, my Brand, and Mer-awareness, becoming a brand ambassador for a few different brands, a professional Merman, and an underwater model, and allowing me to showcase products. I can show the world how to "look cool underwater' – let me show you!

Social media platforms are positive; it's my best business card and an ever-evolving space like the ocean. The entertaining content I can share wholeheartedly and express my aquatic conservation vision, learn more about my customers, and also gather new leads. Posting an informal caption, I subconsciously teach people to do the right thing in nature—A space of influence. I can see it now, as it happened in Fort Lauderdale; Teens and children will call out adults and Parents after dropping a bag or littering to the beach, "The Mermaids will see you!!" —that matters most, holding people accountable.

If I feel like I'm having a bad day, or I see someone else having a bad day, I POSE; that one smile or giggle I get back, maybe that could change the entire day. "Hi, how are you?" I say. Pose ready!

Growing up, a phrase I used to say often was, "You only die once," I've now swapped that to "You only live once. You live every day, die one time….. Live it". It all can be taken away so quickly. I've watched how quickly the water can take it away. A mask I was using in the ocean one day was swept away; I felt the fear that day; I could have been swept away too, but now I live it – the fear–embrace everything that scares me, and go for it.

I free myself when I perform to be the fabulous me and emotionally move into new glorious experiences. I honor myself by asking for what I want. Visit me at mermanandrew.com

Mermaids don't care about the opinions of shrimp!

Have a Mer-mazing day!

If you can't find me, could you check the caves?

About the Author

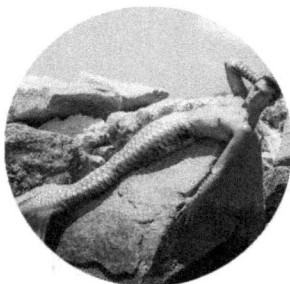

Merman Andrew Corter is a public figure based in Florida, USA. He has created a Mer-mazing business brand and career as a professional Merman utilizing his experience in performing arts, corporate settings, ambassadorship, modeling, entertainment, and all things aquatic. He embodies his profession with innate qualities in BECOMING his Mer-self with pride and passion.

Highly passionate about Marine Conservation and aquatic awareness and charity work, spreading inclusion, and developing new skills. He is changing the world, one smile and wave at a time. As the water beacons him, all negativity is lost; He may even grant you a wish with his gorgeous fin swish.

If you find him—be SHORE to say SHELLO!

Instagram: Andrew Corter (@mermanandrew) I Instagram
Facebook: https://www.facebook.com/themermanandrew
Tik Tok: @mermanandrew

-ᴡᴡ→

Shay Frost

May we stop seeing ourselves through the eyes of people that never really saw us.

Today I have said THANK YOU to everyone who said I wouldn't amount to anything, had an unfavorable opinion of me, doubted me, was unsupportive, and talked shit. I need to express this from a heart-centered space. One day you will tell your story of overcoming, and this will become someone else's survival guide. These *nay-sayers* have given me the extra drive and motivation to prove myself. When you believe in yourself, it doesn't matter about all the background noise. What matters is your thoughts and feelings; just make sure you work hard and show them by being highly motivated in anything you do! As I say yes to life, life says yes to me. I have learned to appreciate all that I do. I am good enough, just as I am. I speak up for myself. I ask for what I want. I claim my power.

This is just the beginning for me, and I'm so proud of myself, my incredible team, my mentors, and everyone who has supported me. How did I get from my profession as a hairdresser for the past 25 years to an Entrepreneur passionate about shampoo? Yes, Life is fast-paced and hectic, like you, and I love all that too, and by Friday, my hair will be 90% dry shampoo!

A friend said, "You go, girl, You're freakin awesome and inspiring!!!"

Over 85 people also repeated the sentiment on one of my social posts. "F*^ck yeah, look at you now!"

I posted an image of me in my newly presented celebratory blazer as a company founder of my networking business, with both my hands gesturing 'the bird' in victory and communicating my moderate to extreme contempt humorously and playfully. I am seriously laughing in my Cynics' faces. My resilience, discipline, and routine account for getting me places, not my confidence. I have none, yet I'm not shy in my natural professional environment. I know my fortitude will determine my success - never dulling my shine for anyone else. My main life goal is to truly help people, build my empire, level up as a leader, and travel the world selling shampoo.

My daily routine is just that, a consistent routine - with no defaults. I live for my Gym/Fitness and travel. Whether my alarm goes off in those early sparrow-fart hours or not, I'm up and out recharging my soul, a practical way to organize my brain and those vital endorphins flow to set up my day, every day, allowing me to thrive. Strangely the Gym had become my *energetic home*. I never used to be a morning person, as it was never my priority to get out of bed, and I couldn't physically and mentally get out of bed for years. I was lethargic and had a love/hate relationship with the gym as I found it boring and unmotivating, and at times I couldn't stand myself. I eventually called myself out on my mental tracks and excuses and took a personal stand. My challenge in my fitness was creating a 'feeling' within. I had an athletic frame and didn't need to change much. It was all a feeling, not a desired number on the scales. I feel this exact notion has shaped me for success too. 'Don't be a number,' a number society or BMI says you should be. Become a FEELING and a LIFESTYLE consistent with a no-quit attitude in a non-negotiable routine.

Just as important, travelling is not only a change of scenery or an adventure but is a trustworthy source of happiness for me. Bali is my *spiritual home*.

My businesses and work are my *loves*, and it is an unexpectedly close community of incredible humans who have become my friends, team, and future empire. I never knew I needed them before, a close working and energized professional community. Before starting with Network Marketing, I only had a few friends and was always shy until you got to know me. Life got in the way of socializing, and I focused on my family and business rather than personal connections. The genuine friendships I have made while growing my businesses were so unexpected. I initially resonated with the business model and products, but it has been life-changing on so many levels. I had not realized I had been sitting in my comfort zone, and it all seemed like too much effort. I became petrified of meeting new people, and even when I started my businesses, doing video posts, reels, and clips, it sickened me to my core. Fear got in the way. The inner ME stole my tit-bit confidence, but I did it anyway, and lately, others have called me out on being loud and intimidating, clearly now residing in my new confident comfort zone. Ironical.

I share my passion and knowledge for my business daily. I am so animated about the products I work with and promote and the incredible results I've witnessed- I genuinely want to assist everyone, boost their confidence, and nourish their hair and skin. I have seen how these natural products have changed my clients and my family's lives. I have built a fantastic existence for myself, my family, and my team, and I want to assist others in building a business and income stream for themselves. To some people, this may seem 'small.'

I am a salon owner, an accomplished hairdresser, and now an Asia Pacific founder, hosting and presenting Virtual Zoom meetings and events while supporting others.

Recently I found myself enjoying our Last day in Canggu, Bali, back to my spiritual home where my soul gets recharged and nourished. Bali makes my heart happy. Old Man's Smoke House, Brunch Club, and a few others - effectively ate my way around Bali for my 'BIG' 40th birthday!

The day before our last day, we chased the sunrise at Mount Batur Volcano,

With a 2 am start, so much fun and adventure, actual magic. We explored and made memories to cherish for a lifetime. Highly recommend the jeep tours to Mount Batur Volcano in Bali. I want everyone to experience this little adventure at least once.

Next? Off to the USA in September 2023 for our company's annual convention- LIVING THE DREAM.

My passion for work and business as an entrepreneur has filled my emotional cup, watching my team grow and celebrating their successes.

My salon work and network marketing go hand in hand; I help with hair and scalp concerns, educating clients in making better-informed choices regarding haircare and skincare with tips on making them feel more confident about themselves.

I'm a mother and wife (I sometimes feel strict and rigid), and like you, I juggle life's stresses. It's my personality to KEEP IT REAL in our household. I don't like "fluff" and carry-on. I banter back and forth with our boys, our high achiever's sons; one is academic, and the other is sports scholarship. Highly moralistic and proud parents is an understatement. We encourage them to be the best version of themselves.

Ben has always been supportive of everything I do. He has been my biggest fan since, and now he gets VIP customers so I can *retire him so he can become a "Mo-Man!"* (The other hubbies have this tagline). Strike a Pose.

Enter the controversy regarding direct sales and network marketing.

It's an exciting thought - Regardless of people's opinions of how one feels about Network Marketing and Direct Sales:

You don't buy supplements/haircare/skincare from **your friend** in direct sales primarily for fear of specific schemes, BUT you buy from large chain stores with shelves full of harmful products…ummmmm…because…because why? It's where you buy things, right? The stores.

Wait, who *are* you supporting?

When you buy haircare or skincare from a large chain store, you are helping the big wigs add to their top-line value of billions of dollars.

The direct sales market is growing, and more and more 'everyday' people are looking for alternative ways to make money!

When you purchase from your friends, you are helping buy groceries, pay bills, or repair the car. YOU are helping a family gain financial security, pay their rapidly increasing mortgage, save for retirement, and to help with University costs. YOU are assisting a Mum to relieve the financial burden, putting money towards a family trip, and funding the kid's annual sporting activities. ☺You also get quality products with fantastic customer service!

Shop small businesses - yeah, that includes direct sales and affiliate programs!

This small business 'Mums' appreciate your support more than you may realize.

Behind the Chair

I have been in this industry as a hairdresser for over 25 years.

It was my passion for so long, but being such a demanding, tiring job, it became just a JOB, something I had to do to make money each week to pay the bills. I wasn't happy. I became bored and hated walking into the salon. I encourage health and wellness in our household, but chocolate is an exception.

As a kid, I was shy but loved my own company. Becoming a hairdresser gave me the space to bring forth a creative side. I now love going to events and sharing stories with people.

In October 2021, I partnered with a new vegan, non-toxic haircare company, which has changed my life! I never knew that shampoo would have such an impact on my life in so many ways.

Firstly let's just address that still, to this day, I'm shocked at the fantastic results I see and experience daily from these products. Secondly, I never thought that my passion and purpose would be in helping others with hair/ scalp concerns and trimming; at the time.

I have gone from working full time, 12 hr days, six days a week, missing out on family events, and so much more.

I have successfully cut back by 1/2 of b*ehind-the-chair* but have increased my income and helped so many others build a successful online businesses that they can call their own and make an income they want around their needs. My passion for the salon has returned, and I love walking into the salon on the days I'm there and helping others every day with this fantastic hair care to build their confidence, which puts a smile on my face.

It's not easy, but let me tell you this, it's the most rewarding and fun time I have ever had. I love everything about it and can't wait for this year to unfold with all my achievements and success.

If you also want more in your life, let's chat and see if you and I would be a good fit to work together! I know that the team community I now have in this biz is something I need and love so much. It's the missing link to my professional happiness.

Two thousand twenty-three big things are happening, so you can sit back and watch my journey or be part of the amazing community I have created and love so much!

Team Hairbesties level up!

This Biz is More Than Shampoo

Are you getting results from your purple shampoo? Is your hair still brassy? Let's talk about the color wheel. Brassy tones are yellow/orange on a color wheel, and the opposite side is the purple/blue tones. Pop the purple tone to neutralize those unwanted brassy tones.

Our violet shampoo patented technology illuminates and brighten by going into the inner layers of the hair shaft, not just a topical Product. If you've just spent a small mortgage on getting that desired look and using (please don't tell me) a supermarket brand, you need to invest in yourself. You're worth it.

Hairdressers always taught the products they were to see the professional brands. This is what you are to use and sell as they are best. Boy, was I wrong? I couldn't be more proud to partner with this company. You get nothing but results with the mix of technology and natural ingredients.

Suppose you bought a shampoo | conditioner, and toner from your hairdresser as an after-sales-recommendation.' It's probably because salon reps are making them stock products on shelves to sell.

You don't have to buy it; they might tell you the color won't last if you don't use the matching product.

Our new GLOBALLY released violet shampoo has just launched in Australia, and we are so excited that everyone now has access to it. It's Perfect for bleached hair, blonde hair, brassy brunettes, silver | grey hair, men and women.

As a Market Partner, I have been lucky enough to get my hands on this range early, and I tell you, I'm in love! And so will you.

Thank you so much.

Thank you for choosing to buy your shampoo from me.

Thank you for the support and messages telling me how much you have learned from me.

Thank you for sharing your love of these products with your friends and family. The referrals are life-changing for me.

Thank you for the messages telling me how much confidence you now have again cause you love your hair.

Thank you for trusting me with my recommendations.

Thank you for the new supportive community I have.

Thank you for being a great friend.

Thank you for taking the time to do the things I love and light me up.

Thank you for the encouragement and success I have had.

And most importantly, thank you for your continued support of my passion, purpose, and obsession. I want you to know that not only are you supporting me but my whole family, and you have given me a life I once dreamed of that I now live as a reality and get to help others create for themselves.

Thank you from the bottom of my heart.

Straightening Crowns

I sit at The Grand Hyatt, Nassau City, in the Bahamas. The "Bahama Mammas" are besties who work and travel together. No more than 12 hrs working days each week in my salon. Yes, Good things are coming!

As I sit here in the Bahamas and reflect on how far I have come, I genuinely need to pinch myself. I'm hard on myself sometimes, but that's just my nature always to want to do & be better.

I have worked so hard these last 12 months that it has led me to October. Here, I had a MASSIVE life-changing goal, with three days and a few hours left to get there.

DON'T EVER GIVE UP ON YOURSELF!

To everyone out there that supports me, I can't thank you enough. Like I always say, when you buy shampoo from me, you support my whole family and change our lives, and I will always be thankful. I am grateful that we stand out from the rest!

Dermatologically and ophthalmologically tested.

Vegan, plant-based ingredients, non-toxic and gluten-free. They were leaping bunny certified.

Naturally-based formulas produce tangible results that are all proven and tested.

Our Scientific Advisory Board developed it in-house—a panel of specialists who confirm all science, clinical, and formulation.

I don't know about you, but I want it to work and deliver results if I pay for something.

What do you use on your body?

Skin•vest•ment

(Noun)

Take action and invest time into your skin routine to achieve healthy, glowing, and supple skin. Invest in products with natural ingredients that work.

All our products are plant-based anti-aging ingredients, vegan & gluten-free. We are proud to be leaping bunny approved!

My new rules for wellness? Passion is energy. Feel the power that comes from focusing on what excites you! Be loud and talk about the things that are important to you. Connect with me, and let's chat about your hair and Skin-vestment!

We all are intrinsically like books; I resonate as a published author. Most people only view the cover, the minority read only the introduction, and many more believe the critics as the wildfire of innuendo and gossip run free. Only some people will know our full valuable content.

If you don't make time for wellness, a forced time off to address your Illnesses arrives—time to construct your survival guide. Life happens for you, not to you, so learn to pick your lip up and get shit done because no one will do it for you.

Claim your power.

About the Author

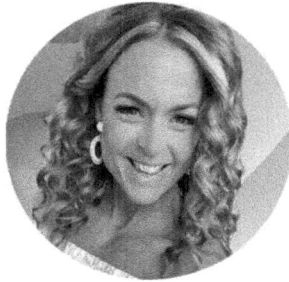

Shay Frost is a real powerhouse woman: Entrepreneur, Hair Care Specialist, owner and operator of the Head Shed Hairdressing Mackay, and a leader in her network marketing company for naturally based anti-aging hair and skin care products.

She resides with her husband and two boys in Mackay, Queensland, Australia.

Shay is passionate about supporting local businesses, offering timeless health advice for hair and skin care, travels regularly, and loves a good Prada handbag.

"Every woman's success should be an inspiration to another"
- Shay Frost.

Website: shayfrost.mymonat.com
Instagram: @shayfrosty
Facebook: https://www.fabebook.com/shay.frost

-ww→

Lord John Hacking

I am living a high life with the distinguished title of Lord Hacking.

The Proclamation reads:

"On the Twenty-First of May in the year of two thousand and twenty-one, on the sixtieth year of rein of our sovereign lady Elizabeth the Second, by the grace of God, of the United Kingdom of Great Britain and North Ireland and her other realms and territories Queen, Head of Commonwealth, Defender of Faith, delivered unto us the intention bequeath Lord unto the dedication of land in Scotland in Wigtownshire. Henceforth and in perpetuity be known by the style and title Lord John Hacking"

Hidden deep in the picturesque Scottish Sub-Kingdom Medieval Lordship of West Galloway lies one-of-a-kind Lord and Lady titles once reserved for the blue-blooded. From the majestic town square and Councils meeting place on Lewis Street to the Galloway whisky distilleries, stunning wild scenery, and of course, Loch Ryan bordering the Irish Sea, as the crow flies to the Isle of Man–which you can see on a clear day. Brushing past wildlife-filled wetlands and sweeping hills dotted with ruined castles is just the beginning. Learn of myths and legends as you journey between Scotland's jagged peaks. Scotland is that no matter where you find yourself, a castle is never far away. Some grand estates allow an incredible stay in their historic rooms, a fortress with sumptuous interiors and outstanding views.

Wigtownshire's western "hammer-head," its small rock islands, and its many ferries from Scottland to Northern Ireland are being watched by the Mull of Galloway Lighthouse and Wigtown castle.

I would happily be called Lord of the Castle—extending 5 stories high, pool and gymnasium, and the most comfortable lounge and bar. I am sitting here with 13-year-old Glengrant Single Malt Scotch in my crystal tumbler with large "W" shaped ice cubes— the lord of my castle here in Australia. An American with a Scottish Lord title, living in Australia.

My historic roots initially took me to Germany, then to the USA. I am from a hard-working Mom and Dad Military family; my childhood involved travel and relocating many times; I was considered a "military brat" and lived in multiple states. We threw roots in Washington State, the longest we stayed in one state, so plant we did.

As a young man, I was asked what I wanted to be. Blissfully happy, I replied.

Another question only a few years ago; what would you be if you had all the time and money? Similar answer—Be blissfully happy and the kind of my castle.

People have told me," You won't amount to anything." Yea, hard times hit for some long years. The ridicule continued. I tried to find my bliss in many places.

My New Rule for wellness: you can be anything you want to be, even if you feel you have seen better days. If you put your mind to it, you can do what you wish to self-belief can create a life you never imagined.

One day in late 2015, I packed a suitcase, passport in hand, and jumped on an Air New Zealand flight to Australia with my now-wife, Dee. She rescued me, and I rescued her. My little bag of clothing was more than I needed to travel the world, I needed bliss and love, and I persevered with my residency applications.

Was it all easy?

Coming to Australia was a lifestyle change and creating a life we love. Significant challenges come with great goals, but it's your reactions to them and how you carry yourself out of the gold. As Cash is King, Goals are Queen, and Bliss is Trump. Like playing a hand of cards,

"Each player must accept the card's life deals, but once they are in hand, he alone must decide how to play the cards to win the game."

I am a fan of Poker; I have played many games in another life far from here. This is how I learned to pay attention, master myself, and win the game. There is a key to generating new ideas and finding creative solutions to problems. My brain is always busy with new ideas to expand my current thinking. The most prominent bluff is playing my two of spades. Over the years, it's won me many social games. Just as you think you don't have a lot, you may be winning anyway. Making wise and savvy decisions is a recipe for quick thinking, an analytical mind, and bluffing. You don't choose the hand you are dealt. Understanding the game's complexity, as in life, hopefully, you can turn to your advantage. Just like life, every situation is different. We have created many experiences in Australia far beyond my childhood image of BLISS.

Snorkeling on The Great Barrier Reef. Speed boating out on a giant inflatable craft, Ocean Rafting (if you are ever up this way in Airlie Beach- I highly recommend the trip to Whitehaven Beach), plunging into the crystal warm waters; the coral colors vibrant, the fish inquisitive, and a 6ft long Blue Humphead

Maori Wrasse with thick lips, a white-tip-reef shark gently gliding past the small rock aperture. Fish pellets were scattered on the surface of the waves by giggling tour operators, and a hundred flapping fins and gaping mouths ascended on top of us; many screams were heard...Bliss, it was for me.

Fishing trips in the Whitsunday waters are just as magical as the life we have created.

Fishing provides such peace— true relaxation and fun for the sport of it all. The catch and release philosophy, many different species, catching a Red Emperor 2/3 my body size–I'm over six and a half feet tall; such a highlight! The Oceans force took over that day, rough seas and so many harsh wave crashes, and the boat launched its bow, where we could hardly stand and couldn't walk, angry storms arising, scaring the life out of us and the reality you reach—- you are who you are. Anything can happen at any time in 3-meter swells and lighting strikes. Don't let it stop you. We are all stuck in some way, don't let your circumstances or associates or lack of inspiration- not even yourself. Be your own worst enemy or your greatest advocate.

Our life is filled with surprises, like getting a selfie what a Kangaroo on Cape Hillsborough beach. The native animals graze at sunrise on the beach and dig for roots.

Snowboarding in Queenstown, New Zealand, placing a padlock of love on bridges at the boardwalk with my beautiful wife, and planning to return to see if our padlock is still there.

Celebrating my 50th birthday in Surfers Paradise, Australia, knocking shoulders with USA Musical Royalty, and staying for a week at the Hilton Hotel.

SIppig cocktails in airports worldwide because we can, from Portland to Los Angeles, Arizona, New York to New Zealand, Australia, and Fiji, and where next?

All Bliss!

A more incredible Bliss than I ever imagined.

Second Rule of Wellness; you need to learn to enjoy the game. Rare doesn't mean impossible. Do different things, random things, off-the-cuff things, who cares? Start a business, fail, and start over. Don't like it, get out! You're not a quitter; just choosing what life you want to lead, right? You show your greatness by the hands you fold, not the hands you play.

The books of Warren Buffett inspire me. For years wanting to start my own business, but now looking from the other side of having those businesses and company we built, yet realizing that was not what I wanted. Yet inspiration comes in many forms.

'The Warren Buffet Way,' "The Life Lessons & Rules For Success,' and ' Ground Rules' offer insight into a man who started with nothing multi-billionaire. Did it let anybody talk him down? I love his ideology that 'Someone is sitting in the shade today because someone planted a tree a long time ago.' We are now reaping the rewards of planting our trees years ago. The chains of habit most of my life have been too tight to be felt and heavy to be broken in my past; bliss has broken them away and renewed my life completely.

'Should you find yourself in a chronically leaking boat, devoting the energy-changing vessels is more likely to be more productive than patching leaks.'

Dee and I have changed trajectory and time to arrive at where we are now. The ability to travel, visit countries, and choose what we fill our day with - bliss.

It's interesting one's own family and friends can influence you one way or the other- my parents were supportive, unlike many of my friends. Trouble became them. I am so grateful for having the ultimate family support when moving to Aus to realize my dream and potential in my business and Hacking Enterprises company successfully. Owning multiple businesses in a short time resonates with the struggle of a start-up and what it takes to do it all; I can't imagine what Mr. Buffet went through.

Imagine being told 30 years ago your then-girlfriend, who you fell in love with, would return to Australia after her 12-month student exchange year and come back and collect you for a better life. She did, although being 28 yrs later. I am grateful; a couple of heartbreaks later, a fantastic Son after, lots of ridiculousness and 'boy behavior' (got all that out of the way), life lessons learned to live our blissful state now together, and now a loving extended family who I love with all my heart–now so blessed with a granddaughter.

Life is not a matter of always holding good cards but of playing a poor hand well!

I was so elated to receive the distinguished title of Lord Hacking as a birthday gift—a patch of land purchased in Scotland. I have finally become the Lord of the Castle—extending 5 stories high, our apartment complex in Mackay, Queensland; we have that pool and gymnasium I imagined and the most comfortable lounge and bar in our gorgeous apartment. I feel like I am the Mayor of Alfred Street, working within the complex and feeling very at home with my pretty Lady. Lord and Lady living a blissful life. We love our large fortress: no castellated turrets, winding spiral staircases, and a bottle-necked dungeon. Explore the grounds, but is a home for my Clan—a fort with a sumptuous interior and outstanding views.

This evening, I am sitting here with 13-year-old Glengrant Single Malt Scotch in my crystal tumbler with large "W" shaped ice cubes—the lord of my castle. We will get to Wigtownshire's great land one day, exploring Scotland, Dee's family heritage, and our plot of land. The Lord and Lady titles, once reserved for the blue-blooded – are now available to the public for the first time!

Purchased our Scottish Title Pack directly and gave us the ultimate gift!

I am Lord Hacking. Blissfully happy—— blissfully satisfied as Lord of my castle.

About the Author

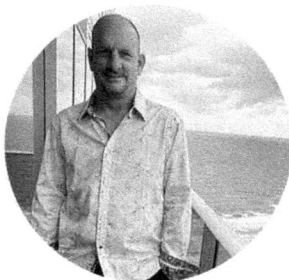

Lord John Hacking sips his Scotch Galloway Single Grain Whisky perched in his plush Oaken chair, presiding over his Castle in Far North Queensland, Australia, living his merry life with his loving wife, three kids abroad, and one gorgeous granddaughter in his hometown Spokane, Washington, USA.

He was a former Entrepreneur and company owner, now a property investor, and assisted his mates in their business wherever possible.

Play every hand; you can't miss them all.

Facebook: www.facebook.com/johnhacking
Email: johnhacking@gmail.com

-ᴡᴡᐅ

Malik Hayat

Unleashing your potential is a powerful and transformative endeavor that involves tapping into your unique talents, abilities, and strengths to achieve extraordinary outcomes. It is the process of unlocking the dormant capabilities within you and embracing the limitless possibilities that lie ahead.

To unleash your potential, you must first recognize and understand your worth. Embrace the idea that you are capable of greatness and that your dreams and aspirations are valid. Believe in yourself and develop a strong sense of self-confidence and self-belief.

Next, embark on a journey of self-discovery. Explore your passions, interests, and values to clarify what ignites your soul. Identify your strengths and unique talents and find ways to leverage them in pursuing your goals. Embrace continuous learning and personal development to expand your knowledge and skills and seek opportunities that allow you to grow and evolve.

It is essential to cultivate a growth mindset. Embrace challenges as opportunities for growth, learn from failures and setbacks, and persist in adversity. Embrace change and be adaptable, for it is through adaptation that we thrive in an ever-changing world.

Setting inspiring and meaningful goals is another crucial aspect of unleashing your potential. Define your vision and break it down into actionable steps. Create a plan that includes short-term and long-term goals, and consistently work towards them with focus and determination.

Surround yourself with a supportive network of individuals who believe in you and uplift your spirits. Seek guidance from mentors and role models who have succeeded in areas that resonate with your aspirations.

Unleashing your potential is a transformative journey that requires self-belief, self-discovery, a growth mindset, goal setting, and a supportive environment. Embrace the power within you and embark on a path of personal growth and self-realization. Watch as you surpass your expectations, achieve remarkable things, and lead a life of fulfillment and purpose; this is what I genuinely believe in, and practice it every day of my life; if I can do it, why can't you?

Self-Belief: The Key to Unleashing Your Potential:

Self-belief is fundamental in unleashing your potential. It is the unwavering faith and confidence in your abilities, worth, and potential for success. Without self-belief, even the most exceptional talents and skills may remain dormant and underutilized. In contrast, with a strong self-belief, you can overcome obstacles, embrace challenges, and achieve remarkable feats. This chapter explores the importance of self-belief and provides strategies to cultivate and strengthen it.

The Power of Self-Belief:

Self-belief acts as a catalyst for personal growth and achievement. When you genuinely believe in yourself, you become more willing to take risks, explore new opportunities, and step outside your comfort zone. It fuels your motivation, determination, and resilience in adversity. With self-belief, you develop a positive mindset that empowers you to embrace challenges as stepping stones to success rather than insurmountable barriers.

Self-belief also influences how you perceive and interpret setbacks. Rather than viewing failures as reflections of your worth or abilities, you see them as valuable learning experiences and opportunities for growth. This mindset shift allows you to bounce back stronger, adapt your approach, and persist in pursuing your goals.

Cultivating Self-Belief:

Building self-belief is a journey that requires conscious effort and practice. Here are some strategies I practice to develop and strengthen my self-belief.

Challenge Limiting Beliefs:

Identify and challenge any limiting beliefs undermining your self-belief. Replace negative self-talk and self-doubt with positive affirmations and empowering thoughts. Recognize that your past does not define your future and that you have the potential to achieve greatness.

Celebrate Past Achievements:

Reflect on your accomplishments, no matter how small they seem. Celebrate your successes and acknowledge the skills, qualities, and efforts that contributed to them. This reflection reinforces your belief in your abilities and reminds you what you can achieve.

Surround Yourself with Positivity:

Surround yourself with positive influences and supportive individuals who uplift and encourage you. Seek mentors, friends, or family members who believe in your potential and provide constructive feedback and guidance. Minimize exposure to negative influences or individuals who undermine your self-belief.

Visualization and Affirmations:

Engage in visualization exercises where you vividly imagine yourself achieving your goals and living up to your potential. Use positive affirmations to reinforce your self-belief. Repeat statements that affirm your worth, abilities, and potential, such as "I have what it takes to succeed."

Set Realistic Goals and Celebrate Progress:

Set realistic goals that align with your values and aspirations. Break them down into manageable steps and track your progress. Celebrate each milestone and use these successes as evidence of your capabilities, further strengthening your self-belief.

Embrace Self-Compassion:

Treat yourself with kindness, understanding, and forgiveness. Embrace self-compassion by acknowledging that setbacks and mistakes are a natural part of growth. Practice self-care and prioritize your well-being; a healthy and balanced mindset contributes to overall self-belief.

Continuous Learning and Skill Development:

Invest in continuous learning and skill development. Acquire knowledge and develop skills relevant to your goals and aspirations. The more expertise and competence you gain, the more confident you become in your abilities, bolstering your self-belief.

Take Action and Embrace Challenges:

Take consistent action towards your goals, even if it means stepping into the unknown or facing uncertainty. Embrace challenges as opportunities for growth and view them as valuable experiences that contribute to your personal development. Each time you overcome a challenge, your self-belief strengthens.

Let self0belief propel you, enabling you to overcome obstacles, embrace challenges, and achieve remarkable feats. Strategies include challenging limiting beliefs, celebrating past achievements, surrounding yourself with positivity, and visualization, setting realistic goals, embracing self-compassion, continuous learning, and taking action to empower yourself to unlock your true potential. Believe in yourself, trust your abilities, and believe in your journey. Remember, you are capable of achieving greatness.

Building Habits: The Key to Consistency and Success

Habits are the building blocks of our lives, shape our daily routines and actions, and ultimately determine our level of success. Building positive habits is essential for achieving long-term goals and creating a fulfilling life. As I always tell myself, "Winning is a habit, not an option." This quote emphasizes the importance of cultivating habits that lead to success. Let's discuss and explore the significance of building habits and provide practical strategies to develop positive habits.

The Power of Habits:

Habits profoundly impact our lives because they operate on autopilot, shaping our behaviors and outcomes. Positive habits create a framework for success, consistency, and personal growth, streamlining actions, eliminating decision fatigue, and helping us focus on our priorities. Building positive habits creates a solid foundation for achieving our goals and unleashing our true potential.

Identify Core Values and Goals:

Start by clarifying your core and long-term goals. Align habits with these values and plans to make them meaningful and purposeful. What truly matters to you becomes more sustainable and motivating.

Start Small and Be Consistent:

Begin with small, achievable habits that are easy to integrate into your daily routine. Consistency is vital—a time frame of 21 days to establish a solid foundation. Gradually increase the difficulty or intensity.

Make it Specific and Measurable:

Clearly define the habit and make it specific and measurable. For example, instead of saying, "I will exercise more," specify the pattern as "I will exercise for 30 minutes every morning." This clarity helps you track progress and stay accountable.

Set Triggers and Reminders:

Create triggers or cues that prompt you to engage in the habit. It could be a specific time of day, a visual reminder, or linking the habit to an existing routine. Use technology or tools like alarms, calendar reminders, or habit-tracking apps to keep you accountable.

Accountability and Support:

Share your habit-building journey with a trusted friend, family member, or accountability partner. Having someone to report progress to and receive support can significantly enhance your commitment and motivation.

Track Progress and Celebrate Milestones:

Use a habit tracker or journal to record your daily efforts. Celebrate milestones to reinforce your sense of achievement and motivate further progress.

Be Mindful of Setbacks and Adjustments:

Acknowledge that setbacks are a natural part of habit-building. If you slip up, don't let it discourage you. Instead, view setbacks as opportunities to learn and make adjustments to improve your approach. Reflect on setbacks and modify your strategy accordingly.

Focus on Self-Discipline and Willpower:

Self-discipline and willpower and needed for the building process. Cultivating these traits is essential to practicing self-control, setting boundaries, and prioritizing goals. The habit becomes more manageable and requires less conscious effort.

I believe "Winning is a habit, not an option." By intentionally developing practices that align with your values and goals, you create a solid foundation for personal growth and achievement.

Remember to start small, be consistent, and make your habits specific and measurable. Set triggers, track progress, and seek support to stay accountable and embrace setbacks with self-discipline, willpower, and commitment; you will unlock the power of consistency and propel yourself toward success.

Taking Risks and Making Change: Embracing Opportunities for Growth and Transformation

I always try to jump for the moon; growth and transformation often require us to step out of our comfort zones, take risks, and embrace change—our potential to discover new possibilities through these courageous acts and create a life of fulfillment and purpose. I will explain the importance of taking risks and making change, providing insights and strategies to help you navigate uncertainties and reap the rewards beyond your comfort zone.

The Power of Taking Risks:

An essential component of personal growth and achieving extraordinary outcomes–risks.

It involves stepping into the unknown, facing fears, and challenging the status quo. Taking calculated risks opens us to new opportunities, experiences, and perspectives, pushing our comfort zone boundaries and fostering resilience, adaptability, and self-confidence.

Breaking free from the limitations that keep us stagnant and embracing growth. Risks provide valuable learning experiences, even if unexpected outcomes allow lessons from failures and refine our strategies for future endeavors. Taking risks often leads to incredible rewards and opportunities that we may not have encountered otherwise.

Embracing Change:

Change is an inherent part of life and is crucial for personal growth and transformation. Change presents new possibilities, challenges, and perspectives—evolve, adapt, and explore untapped potential.

Its tarts with openness and curiosity. Recognize that change brings opportunities for learning, growth, and self-discovery. Rather than resisting or fearing change, approach it with excitement and a willingness to explore uncharted territories.

Strategies for Taking Risks and Making Change:

Clarify Your Vision and Goals: Clarify your vision and identify goals that align with your values and aspirations. A clear direction provides a sense of purpose motivating you.

Assess the Potential Risks and Rewards: Before taking a risk or changing, evaluate the risks and rewards involved. Consider the potential benefits, challenges, and potential outcomes. Assessing the risks allows you to make informed decisions and take calculated risks that have the potential for a positive impact.

Step Out of Your Comfort Zone: Growth lies outside your comfort zone. Challenge yourself. Start with small steps and gradually increase the level of risk or change. You are expanding your horizons and building resilience.

Embrace a Growth Mindset: Adopt a growth mindset that embraces challenges—view failures as opportunities for learning and growth. Believe your abilities and intelligence can be raised through effort and perseverance.

Plan and Prepare: Research, gather information, and arm yourself with knowledge—while taking risks and making a change involves a degree of uncertainty, it's essential to plan and prepare as much as possible. Having a well-thought-out plan provides a sense of security and confidence.

Seek Support and Collaboration: Surround yourself with a supportive network of individuals who encourage and believe in your ability to take risks and make change. Mentors, coaches, or peers with experience in the areas you're venturing into—don't be shy to ask for help and honor others' opinions. Collaboration and support can provide guidance, advice, and a sense of reassurance.

Learn from Setbacks and Adapt: Setbacks and challenges may arise when taking risks or making changes. Instead of letting them deter you, view setbacks as learning opportunities—resilience, adaptability, and analysis are essential qualities that allow you to navigate obstacles and continue moving forward.

Cultivate Self-Reflection and Self-Compassion: Engage in self-reflection while taking risks and making change—assess your progress, celebrate achievements, and identify areas for improvement. Additionally, practice self-compassion by being kind and understanding toward yourself during times of uncertainty or setbacks–it's a journey; growth takes time.

Personal growth and transformation do achieve remarkable outcomes. You unlock new opportunities and expand your horizons by stepping out of your comfort zone, embracing change, and adopting a growth mindset. Remember to clarify your vision, assess risks, plan and prepare, seek support, learn from setbacks—and align with your true self.

Be a Hustler: Don't Rest Until You Win

Welcome to the world of hustlers! We're here to shake things up, break the mold, and show you how to unleash your inner go-getter. It's time to wear your hustler hat, buckle up, and prepare for a wild ride toward success. So grab some popcorn because this will be one heck of an adventure!

The Hustler Mindset:

Unwavering Determination: Picture a bulldog with its jaws locked onto a bone. That's the kind of determination we're talking about. Hustlers have a fire burning inside them that can't be extinguished. They set their sights on their goals and don't let anything or anyone stand in their way. They're like bulldozers, bulldozing through obstacles and leaving a trail of success in their wake.

Relentless Work Ethic: Hustlers work harder than a squirrel gathering nuts for Winter. They put in the hours, sweat, and tears to make things happen. They're the Energizer Bunnies of the success world, never running out of battery. While others are chilling on the couch, hustlers are grinding, hustling, and making things move.

Goal-Oriented: Hustlers are like heat-seeking missiles locked onto their targets. They know exactly what they want and go after it with a laser focus. They break their goals into bite-sized chunks and tackle them individually. It's like a game of Pac-Man, gobbling up achievements and leveling up along the way.

Resilience in the Face of Challenges: Hustlers are like rubber bands. No matter how much they're stretched, they always bounce back. They embrace challenges like a thrill-seeking adventurer, knowing that each obstacle is an opportunity for growth. They're not afraid to get knocked down because they know they'll get up even more robust.

Self-Motivation: Hustlers are their cheerleaders, coaches, and fans. They immediately get someone to pat them on the back or give them a gold star. They have an internal fire that keeps them going, pushing them to do their best daily. They're like human tornadoes, generating their motivation wherever they go.

Continuous Learning: Hustlers are knowledge junkies. They have an insatiable thirst for learning and improving. They devour books, podcasts, and courses like a hungry hippos. They know that the more they learn, the more they grow, and the closer they get to their dreams. They're like sponges, soaking up wisdom and expanding their horizons.

Embrace Challenges as Opportunities: Hustlers see challenges as exciting puzzles waiting to be solved. They don't run away from difficulties; they run towards them with open arms. It's like a roller coaster ride, full of twists and turns that keep them on their toes. They're thrill-seekers, always up for an adventure.

Persistent and Tenacious: Hustlers never give up, even when the going gets tough. They're like bulldogs with a bone (again!). They keep pushing forward, no matter how often they stumble or fall. They're the superheroes of persistence, refusing to accept defeat.

Embodying the Hustler Mentality:

Set Clear Goals: Think of your goals as treasure maps leading to buried treasure. The clearer your goals, the easier it is to find that treasure. So, grab your map and start charting your course to success!

Develop a Strong Work Ethic: Work hard, play hard. That's the motto of a hustler. Roll up your sleeves, dive into your tasks, and give it your all. Remember, success loves a hardworking hustler.

Embrace Challenges: Challenges are like thrilling roller coasters. Strap yourself in, scream at the top of your lungs, and enjoy the ride. Embrace the twists and turns because they're the moments that make you stronger.

Learn from Failures: Failure is just a detour, not a dead-end. Treat each failure as a valuable lesson. It's like a secret weapon that prepares you for future battles. So fail, learn, and conquer.

Surround Yourself with Like-Minded Hustlers: Find your tribe of hustlers. Surround yourself with people who lift you, inspire you, and share your hustle mentality. It's like having a squad of cheerleaders cheering you on.

Stay Focused and Disciplined: Avoid shiny object syndrome and focus on your goals. Be disciplined with your time, prioritize your tasks, and slay your to-do list like a boss. You've got this!

Take Action: Action is the secret sauce of hustlers. It's the fuel that powers your dreams. So stop dreaming and start doing. Take that leap of faith and make things happen.

Being a hustler is like being the star of your blockbuster movie.

It's about embracing challenges, working hard, and never settling for less. So buckle up, put on your hustler hat, and get ready for the ride of your life. Remember, you're the hero of your story, and success is waiting for you at the end of the rainbow. So go out there, be a hustler, and don't rest until you win! Unleashing your potential, believe in yourself, and Let the adventure begin!

I will conclude my chapter with a saying by the famous poet from Pakistan, Dr. Allama Iqbal wrote:

خُودی کو کر بُلند اتنا کہ ہر تقدیر سے پہلے

خُدا بندے سے خُود پوچھے بتا تیری رضا کیا ہے

"Elevate yourself so high that even God, before issuing every decree of destiny, should ask you: Tell me, what is your intent?"

About the Author

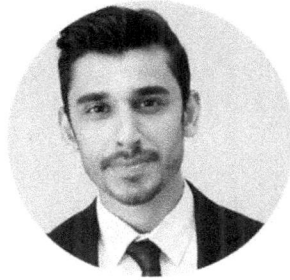

Malik was born in Pakistan into a political family, where the political landscape shaped his early years. Tragedy struck, leaving his younger brother and himself under the care of their courageous and resilient mother (Shahida Bano), who raised her boys as a single mother. Malik embarked on a journey of self-discovery and personal growth, which led me to Australia. He pursued higher education in business, equipping himself with the knowledge needed to succeed.

Through perseverance and determination, he found a calling in the hospitality industry. He is now the Area General Manager for Minor Hotels, overseeing the management of five hotels in Central Queensland, Australia. His journey from humble beginnings to becoming a successful hotelier is a testament to the power of hard work, resilience, and the unwavering support of his family, and is grateful for the opportunities.

LinkedIn: Malik Hayat | LinkedIn
Email: malik_hayat@outlook.com
Instagram: Instragram-Malik_Hayat

-MM->

Dr. Hollywood - ANON.

"I have had dreams, and I have had nightmares, but I have conquered my nightmares because I have dreams"
-J.Salik

Everything that irritates us about ourselves can be a validation to address what is within; skin deep, brain deep, and permission-of-self-deep. During my medical career, I have found it surprising that a thoughtful quote or a personal transformational journey can inspire others; I now live in limitless love, light, and joy. All is well, and health is wealth for myself and my patients. It wasn't always this way, and in a true sense, my journey to Hollywood has been paved with drama. Ironically, Hollywood is the home of dramatic energy, yet I don't like drama. If you had told that little boy from Kuwait that he would be a Doctor living in California, changing people's lives, he would have stared back at you blankly, kicking the dirt and stones with his big toe in the family kitchen. That little boy is now a man in his prime, creating peacefulness of mind for others, the sanctuary of body, and reflecting health. We must start somewhere and have somewhere to go; the journey, not the destination, provides joy.

Joining the celebrity plastic surgeons in Hollywood initially was a business strategy for me. From Kuwait to Sydney, Australia, to study medicine. The USA was only on my radar once I was approached. Also, did I ever see myself appearing on one episode of The Celebrity Plastic Surgeons of Beverly Hills show? Incomprehensible! Now living in my West Hollywood compound, my celebrity enclave, close to all that matters to me, my family, and my work. My wife, Mother, and Brother have all taken up residence, and we have a little boy of our own on the way—so many reasons to celebrate.

The human body and form are to be celebrated, and being a part of an integral team that accomplishes this is life-changing and rewarding work. Specialising in transformation surgery and a specialist plastic surgeon in cosmetic procedures, Gender-affirming surgery, and form-of-body reconstruction significantly improve quality of life. In my own experiences of improving my health and function of my body, the self-esteem of appearance, and self-confidence. Do we, not all, deserve to seek and gain happiness by living life, being confident within our bodies we build and hope, so social anxiety I suffered becoming a new surgeon in the field and committing to my physical health. This undoubtedly is what brought me to Hollywood to build my current existence.

The urban fringe of Kuwait is my hometown; when I was a child, children faced hunger, malnutrition, exploitation, and loss of education; we were sad, worried, and scared. I was fortunate to have left my remote community (devoid of a permanent health clinic) for Australia, the land of opportunity. I vowed to become a Doctor after being exposed to many situations. Life was far less challenging for our family, and I was fortunate to be offered the chance to study at Australia's top medical University.

Again, so fortunate to be associated with an innovative Faculty of Surgeons in a dynamic and complex arena. I secured a leading role that ensured a specialist plastic surgeon residency and gained my RACS, USA registration via ABPS with a further 6 years of training. My introduction to California was crucial for my career, relocating my family, and meeting my now wife, all in the first month of emigrating to America. It soon became apparent that private practice was best suited, and as a 'Celebrity Surgeon' have made a name for myself. Board-certified by the American Board of Plastic Surgery and aligned with other renowned surgeons who have performed over 25,000 procedures. Extreme Makeover show came to the forefront of catapulting the industry to a distinguished level—top leaders in aesthetic breast and body surgery.

At this point, the sector changed fast—A more boutique individual approach came forth and more inclined to be inside the client's goals and specific anatomy—not just 'getting surgery rectification.' Safety became the highest priority, which was certainly not in the past. Each procedure is now evaluated by what is best for the patient and putting the patients at ease, yet again a significant change from past practices. The physicians themselves, too, have increased their approachability—warm, friendly, and professional. For many years I had been ridiculed in my field of study, " You're too nice, you will never make it" There was a sentiment of rigidity, 'possibilities' were not to be discovered, and 'Good enough' was not in my vocabulary. I placed love and joy into my work and life for all reasons. I always wanted to feel like I did the utmost for every patient, the best I could do. I love seeing the confidence in women when they are happy with their breast size, shape, and symmetry. My goal is to get the required surgery performed to the desire of my patients, as close to the specific desired result, and the plans for the surgery are of vital importance to me. In addition, it is great to see within the industry that surgeons are working to their credential level, experience, and training. High patient satisfaction rates make or break you in Hollywood. Celebrity clients flock to our clinics as our surgeons are eager to create ' a new them'; their bodies are not where they want them to be, and we can help. I am now highly trained in abdominal liposuction and gynecomastia, such a reaffirming result for the patient's confidence and quality of life.

All healthcare that can reform cannot happen only externally; it must happen inside ourselves, in our external appearance in alignment with who we feel we are, and in our homes, families, and communities. Taking what we do to communities like I grew up in, my area of the Arabian Peninsula is life-reaffirming. Yes, there, too, are clients turning to plastic surgery to satisfy their need for change, regardless of gender. Some Kuwait clients have had 19 surgeries and cosmetic procedures; kidney surgery, facial and airway rectification from fractures, and childhood trauma. Only a few years ago, plastic surgery was almost limited exclusively to women; there has been a shift, and I have moved towards performing medical procedures, life-saving cosmetology, rectifying deformations, and failed surgeries rectification. The demand for skin tightening surgery is rising, as is facial feminization surgery or facial contouring revision, skeletal contouring, and Blepharoplasty.

My experience and time on the Extreme Makeover Documentary series were engaging. I accompanied my colleagues as a backup Surgeon. The sub-culture was kind, but the number of surgeries that had to take place in one location was eye-opening. Joint surgeries and physical deformities are not in my area of expertise. I felt the whole 'mission' was Demonised and rectifying young adults with "ruined lives due to a genetic quirk"---self-esteem shot to pieces, off-the-scale-disproportionate bodies, and radical blossoming due to the surgery seemed quite Sleeping-Beauty-style to me. Advising on the TV shows Gender Dysmorphia Transformation Miracles 'truly extreme,' and 'miracles coming true,' I did not have any surgery time but witnessed the drama. 'Life-saving surgeries' due to a jaw medical condition, Maxillofacial surgery, why are they not on the NHS? Leave it to Extreme Makeover! Ratings?

The desire to feel loved and joyous is universal; I've found my place on the ground in Hollywood, entrenched in our clinical work and my family; I now stay close to home by choice. I didn't like the attention and feel it has hindered me. I feel so close to my family ties and roots; why would I expand my career abroad when I only want to be home? Colleagues will sacrifice anything for more prestige, wealth, and celebrity clientele.

My New Rule for wellness from my perspective—Out of our vulnerabilities will come to our strength. I am safe in my universe, and I love that within my work, I allow safety and comfort for others to live true within their bodies.

As a child, we went as a family to the Gand Mosque in Kuwait City; this trip changed me. I spent at least an hour admiring the architectural beauty, the vastness and luxury inside, and the old Qur'anic manuscript–the most beautiful sanctuary of holiness. I witnessed a group of men in prayer time gathering–disfigured faces all chatting together. I was told 'not to look.' I asked what happened to them; I was told about animal attacks and atrocities as children. Images filled my mind, and I never forgot.

A female patient presented to our clinic years after exploratory surgery due to numerous stab wounds, a long and exasperating battle from injuries sustained from her ex-husband's knife thrusts into her torso and abdomen, but she did not escape unharmed. Her life had been saved, but her scars grew, and a massive incisional hernia and numerous keloid scars developed. Our team performed an incisional hernia repair, multiple scar revisions, abdominoplasty, and liposuction of her flanks. Following her surgery with us, she awoke to a whole new body. Her painful and disfiguring hernia was fixed, and her abdomen returned to its former svelte shape. With the increasing number of polytrauma patients treated at high-level trauma centers, plastic surgery has entered the specialty of traumatology and trauma rectification.

Between January 2022 and December 2022, 5,890 patients with traumatic injuries were admitted to the emergency department of a tertiary hospital. 2,100 patients were hospitalized for surgical treatment and critical care. Among these, 590 patients (35%) required at least one plastic surgery procedure. The patient variables included age, sex, etiology, the injured area, and injury characteristics. We also retrospectively investigated surgical data such as the duration of the operation, hospital stay, length of time from injury to surgery, collaboration with other departments, referral to plastic surgeons, to traumatological specialist treatments.

Having historically completed my time as an integration specialist plastic surgeon in the hospital system contributing to medical science via research, I value the role of plastic surgery in multidisciplinary teams at high-level trauma centers, with referrals to private practice has become increasingly important. The results of these studies may help develop interdisciplinary trauma team strategies and the future workforce required. The face of the plastic surgery industry is changing. I see the change.

THE LINK BETWEEN LOOKING GOOD AND FEELING GOOD.

It wasn't until a dog bite patient that I fully understood this concept–contented and more loving. Victims of dog bite attacks, more often children, suffer severe tissue damage. My young patient required multiple procedures, including plastic reconstructive surgery, tissue expansion, and numerous scar revisions. He had lived with the disfigurement for some years, and his mental health was suffering. He wanted to have a top lip to be able to speak and eat adequately and have the ability to close his right eye. This case was out of the plastic surgical books I read early in my studies. I would look at the graphic photos and say, "Yes, that's what I want to fix!" Bringing joy and freedom back into kids' lives reminded me of the men I saw in the mosque many years before.

I've also noticed my behaviors; my wife and mother make better decisions when in a good mood, after my daily swimming laps, and when I choose exercise over indulgences. When I'm presenting at our clinic with vitality, others around me are vital. As I feel most stable with how I feel I am less likely to be affected by others and their actions. Being comfortable in your skin, looking good for you, honoring your joy, and appreciating and valuing yourself are what life is all about to me.

AFTER THE JOY: You are what you do every day. What do you do? How do you speak about yourself? What's your mental chatter?

I had a Debulking procedure—a procedure where areas of thickened skin are thinned out surgically, along with cartilage grafting— a transfer of cartilage from other sites (ear/rib) to reconstruct the patient's nose. A new man was born after that; you could say he had a signature of outstanding, natural-looking results. I continue to be a perfectionist who takes the time with each procedure until I know the results will be excellent. A colleague of mine had a botched facelift from a previous surgeon, coined a "genius" with facelifts because no one could tell she had had anything done, but people kept telling her how great she looked! When she was asked in an interview with Nightline about what makes him the "go-to surgeon in Hollywood, it's hard to be confronted with yourself at all times!"

The common denominator is that you have conditions that can't be resolved.

They can be. Create dreams out of nightmares. You can conquer!

I want to provide a safe world for my children to grow up in so they are not sad, worried, and scared like I had been—safety and comfort for others to live valid within their bodies.

Bringing joy and freedom into our kids' lives. Out of nightmares come a dream and a world of good habits and self-love = life.

Onward. Upward. Inward.

About the Author

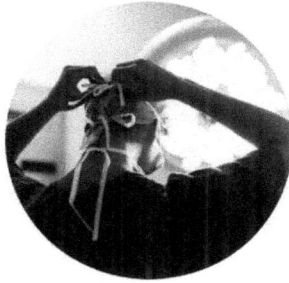

Dr. Hollywood - ANON, an MD F.A.C.S specializing in Cosmetic Surgery and Aesthetic services in Hollywood, California. He contributes to Plastic Surgery Symposiums and prefers to remain anonymous due to Netflix's contractual rights.

When he is not in surgery, speaking on stage, or appearing as a guest for shows, he is swimming laps in his pool and spending invaluable time with his family enjoying the American way of life.

'There is no fun in not being the real YOU'
- Dr. Hollywood.

-vvvv→

Fiona Ireland

"If I get to be me, I belong. If I have to be like you, I fit in."
- Brene Brown.

When we feel the balance within, we can share the best of ourselves.

Gratitude, Peace, and Love were the intentions I set quietly at a beautiful beach on the first sunrise of 2023 with two of my close girlfriends. I also would love others' lives filled with these sentiments, alongside what they desire for themselves.

"Know that the real magic happens when you remember there is always enough, and YOU are always enough." I pulled out a Lion Spirit Oracle card (by Colette Baron-Reid), reminding me that I have a gift of pride and a gentle reminder of self-worth, and this message filled my cup and touched my heart, a space I operate from daily. Belonging in your own skin is being accepted by you. As a skincare specialist, I know being abundant within yourself is a hug for your skin. I support others from my generous heart space. I've learned to traverse the chaos and stresses of life to assist others in expanding themselves. Becoming content in their own skin and being a healthy expression of self can exalt others too. Don't we all want that?

Boss Aesthetics was created from my life's work and my heart.

My clinic offers an array of luxury holistic facials and corrective skin therapies, brow design, cosmetic tattooing, medical tattooing, and gender revision treatments. My vast expertise in my field allows me to deliver exceptional results for my clientele, and daily I feel elevated to connect with people to make a difference. I am so grateful to do this daily work and raise my family. I show my sons and daughter that I can create this life from the ashes of our former life, terrible marriage breakdown, and rise again. I choose to be empowered, sensitive, vital feminine energy, a woman that can leave a legacy and a story with them as they grow and create their own rules for wellness. There has been a prominent feeling around the impact on women to be empowered and strong all the time, and that's OK; it's also OK to be feminine and vulnerable; it's essential to existence. I invite you to think of your rules of wellness.

The Aries in me releases my optimism, strength, and bravery; naturally, a leader in my field, brimming with new ideas, and

I've learned to work with emotional regulation. Within this new reality as a single mother and my self-worth-work, I have developed an awareness and connection of all three bodies; Mental, Emotional, and Physical, driving my clarity of balance. Every moment is transcendent from the space of my beach-sunrise intentions; Gratitude, Peace, and Love. These are the driving forces behind all that I do, and my work in my clinic is a testimony of this, and I'm proud of that. My passions are cosmetic/medical tattooing, scar camouflage tattooing and stretch mark therapy, scaring revision treatments, holistic luxury facials, and corrective skin treatments.

A commitment to great self-work has occurred due to my Divorce, during which it felt like I was set on fire, my life was ablaze, and I couldn't breathe, couldn't see for the thick smoke, and felt there was no way out, coveting my children. Self-esteem and self-worth were at an all-time low; however, I set out to handle this transformation with grace. On the other hand, it felt like I was about to be stepping into a new world of freedom; I felt more in touch with who I became after losing myself, my identity, and my confidence. This is the sentiment of most of my clients (different triggers, of course), but I get them. I get it—to be safe and empowered in our skin. Don't we all want that? To feel safe? Safe should be second nature, like breathing oxygen—a force we all require to survive!

My career in the skin and beauty industry began when I became a Beauty Therapist twenty-eight years ago. I evolved as a Facialist and began to integrate holistic applications. I continued along my career path and had six years working for a Skin Cancer surgeon, learning and developing my skills, knowledge, and expertise, especially with scar therapy and acne. I enjoyed the work more than I realized, and in my clinical practice, I wanted greater control over medical tattooing and holistic facial programs. From my heart space, I got to work. I expanded my holistic facial program, advanced dermal therapies, and skin cancer precaution, integrating and transforming people's skin to what they wanted to change. My favorite question to ask clients is, "What do you want to change about your skin/brows/scarring etc?" Allowing my client to connect to the change or improvements they genuinely desire.

Why have an average facial when you can have an authentic and holistic facial experience?

With a certain quality and luxury around the treatment, a Luxury Holistic Facial is a treatment experience. Overall, yes, we want the results, but we desire connection and the experience of it. We want to experience the JOY, the LOVE, the GRATITUDE behind the event, and the blissful underlying tones. I know I'm not alone when I hop on a website and look at the reviews before making any decisions- we all know what a good and a lousy review entails. Sometimes the difference is the feeling, the care, the passion, the experience.

"Thank You, Fiona, So relaxing; I feel blissfully rejuvenated"
- Jill P.

"Every time I receive a treatment from Fiona, I am blessed with beauty that goes to my soul's core. Her Kahuna facial nurtures and transforms how I see myself - Gratitude." - Jude W.

I connect with my client and hone in on what THEY want, what type of results, and what they could be happier with regarding their skin/body/ailment. We, professionals, see things on a different scale and connect with them on a feeling level. First, people are warriors; then, it becomes a transformational journey. Each client is on their journey, whether it be a gender revision, scar therapy, accident, trauma, medical condition, a cancer journey, menopause, or an ongoing Acne crisis. They must improve their quality of life, confidence, and the desired results. The point of difference is to expect and feel within you, not just assertiveness to a desired clinical outcome.

One gorgeous client has had quite the journey with Breast Cancer:

"Quite a significant journey of breast cancer, a double mastectomy and reconstruction, the final stage was having 3D Areola tattoos so I could feel 'girly' once again. Fiona was brilliant and made the process so

relaxing and exciting. The follow-up was easy, and the outcome was beautiful.

I am so grateful to Fiona and her precision detail, and I am totally in love what the outcome. I recommend Fiona for any tattooing or her treatments, and I will not hesitate to seek her advice for anything else I may need."

#3Dareolatattooclient2021

Reflecting on my childhood and upbringing, it's no surprise that I do what I do, as I used to apply makeup and do fancy nails with my friends when they came to visit. I grew up as an only child, and we would role-play in games of Kings and Queens; I would be concerned for their skin and beauty products, play dress-ups, and later in my teenage years, sketch the human body in life drawing classes with the best charcoal artists can have. I sketched portraits and admired the human form, Anatomy and Physiology, and skin. Even at that young age, my mind gathered the knowledge needed to build on that firm base of human awareness.

The "filling up the tank of enoughness" for me during my adult years was an endless struggle; I seem to embody that now; I AM ENOUGH.

My calmness and decompression valve has always been at the beach. The ocean has a smell; the fresh-salty aromas have a way of eliciting the traumas I experience to float away. The sound of the gentle waves soothe, and the ambiance is a message in itself of tranquility. Time in nature elevates my soul; It's the - aesthetic. The oceanic art of emotionally decompressing releases everything that doesn't serve me; the waves mesmerize me, and I sink my energy and my toes into the sand and feel the connection.

My innate passion extends to my precious family. Raising three teenagers to be highly conscious and high-value sensitive Human beings IS NO EASY FEAT by myself; a single parent I never expected was on the cards. Managing their emotions and have them all tower over me, in their statuesque fashion, "Living in their own vibed mature lives," I find myself echoing, " Who are you, Are you 30 already?" Eye rolls, grunts, and groans seem to be staples in the teenage language. Still, they don't tend to be immune to my Mum-Jokes.

Will my children grow up recalling these fond moments, or rather just see their Mother as surviving and thriving? I've learned the difference between an entire biscuit packet and an empty one, the packets left in the cupboard— *insert eye-roll*

Dear Body: Let me find a way to connect to you and love you:

My Number 1: Keeping skincare simple and bespoke to my clients.

Medical tattooing.

A young client had a traditional laser tattoo removed, and the skin pigment was destroyed and presented as lighter than the surrounding skin. She felt unhappy, affecting her mental well-being. "Let's do something about it!' I completed a scar camouflage procedure. The result was an 80% improvement in blending the surrounding tissues.

Scarring caused by accidents, surgery, laser tattoo removal, stretch marks, and self-harm scars always come back to that invaluable point that, once rectified, feeling good in their skin arrives. Confidence returning is the key to almost everything.

Another young client had an eyebrow issue; she was 13 and had the scar since she was 5. The hair didn't grow back, the teasing at school was unbearable about her half-eyebrow, and once my medical tattoo procedure was completed, 'eyebrow envy' (yes, it's a thing) set in at school. Not only did the teasing stop, but she was blissfully happy, relaxed, and confident with others to be herself again.

It's incredible to facilitate the negative experiences people experience to transform into positive life experiences. The scaring can be a reminder of trauma. The affected skin can be a sign of inward unrest and other health disturbances; it's great to discuss this and highlight possible action plans; it's so different for everyone, every day is different, and it facilitates change.

Acne skin and underlying issues.

Acne can be a real anxiety, irritation, and embarrassment. The biggest villain for acne is leaving the issue either unaddressed or highly medicated.

Teenage and adult acne patients I see regularly either active acne outbreaks or for scaring. Self-esteem and self-worth are common denominators; the face is the first part you share with the world. When this is out of balance, the person feels underrated, treated holistically and individualistically is vital - not a one-size-fits-all application which is the usual orthodox medical method of operation. I work together with each client to find the right journey for them to heal and thrive.

Having suffered from Adult Acne myself in my late 20s and 30s, I uncovered a vast spectrum of intolerances I had to deal with from within. I needed a deep connection with the feelings of trauma and the insecurities that I had gone through. I took all this onboard and expanded my knowledge and health journey into treating conditions and holistic individualistic applications - via self-lessons and learning in my field clinically and personally. I now create my own bespoke treatments and modalities in therapies personalized to each client I treat.

Dear Mind: Let me find an aesthetic that will last space and time.

My other Number 1 is to provide a comfortable, safe space to be you!

Gender Revison Tattoing.

This is one of my ultimate specialties. I offer complete inclusion and a space of comfort. After top surgery, 3D Areola tattooing for all genders, and Bottom surgery for females to males, I create my Phalloplasty tattoo services, offering color and appearance and realistic shape and symmetry with the body. I hold the space, and love, for working with the transgender community providing a customized environment for a safe transition. The skin journey can be prolonged due to hormones changing the skin entirely and scar therapy from surgery.

I continue to create awareness of my services available to the transgender community.

The Aging person.

YES! We are all aging. Since our skin will eventually lose the fight against gravity, let's trump gravity at its own game. Let's get that skin firming, glowing, plump, and luminous and build and retain our collagen. I realize society, in general, always considers Vanity to be a dirty word. When we break it down,

VAIN— is it about feeling good about yourself? Does everyone deserve to feel that way?

I have many 80 and 90-year-old clients. They ask them, "Aren't you too old to have facials? " They reply, "Are you too old to feel good????

My aging clients have sparkle. No more dull skin - naturally radiant at any age. Designer skin solutions for each treatment, Luxury Holistic Facials, and Dermal Therapies. Short-term and long-term maintenance.

Others love my passion for skin integration treatments and holistic facials for aging women and men, especially for skin changes through menopause. We are a little lost at this point in our lives - even medically - there isn't much help other than hormone therapy, and not much else. The community of women needs a connection to their heart space; when our skin is fantastic, we feel a million bucks. When you arrive at being comfortable in your skin, you look beautiful, regardless of anything you may regard as 'flaws.'

Put your trust in the right Skin Therapist who knows her 'shit' (sorry, skin).

I am thriving within my mission to support all genders through their journey with skin conditions, naturally enhancing facial features, and elevating personal acceptance. My attention to detail and exceptional personalized treatment is not only about results but about the experience and supported journey. The Wellness mindset behind loving the skin you are in is where balance and repair meet, inside and outside, holistically. It's OK to be emotional; it's OK to be whatever you are feeling right now. It's OK to be sensitive; it's OK to be human.

Something I feel that set's me apart from others: I lead with a space of integrity. Lead from the heart of authenticity, and love connecting with people. Every one craves to connect in different ways; we all desire to connect; it's a base human need.

Aside from wearing sunscreen daily, our number one anti-aging product, we recommend you find a sunscreen you love. Otherwise, you will only wear it. You need to feel it, love it, smell it. Make 'Skincare Sunscreen' an integral part of your conscious efforts toward your health.

A new rule is BALANCE—a balanced relationship between your head and heart.

We all make so many decisions from the head in life, sucking out all the joy "shouldn't" set in; the word "Selfish" is such a mind F*CK, is never used as a positive thing, "going to be selfish today, and have a facial" such dry words! I'm on a mission to change that.

The New Rule of Wellness: "I'm having a facial today" Because you need this experience in your heart and receive it gratefully. You deserve bloody beautiful skin; Youthful, Dewey, Glowing, and Plump! Create a love of self, not from Ego, but from the heart center; I hope these words jump off the page to you.

I did a treatment for the girls who work with me in Clinic, my Mindfulness Facial, and one struggled to receive. She fought it, but "Yes, I'll do this" eventually, and I delivered the treatment straight from my heart. She sat in this energy space and 'allowed' and could connect with her heart energy too. She admitted that after realizing she had become more disconnected from herself, my facial was a blissful elevation of her body and mind! Yes, this was a skin therapy session, yet FROM THE HEART, connecting straight to heart energy for optimal results - an inner journey just as much as outward healing.

Some life-crashing moments ultimately change you as a person and the trajectory of your mindset forever. I witnessed my Sister and brother-in-law being hurtled into a world of scary with their 2-year-old suffering cardiac arrests multiple times after a rapid decline in his health. Their strength, faith, and intuition saw little Jack, with his VAD Heart, receive a new heart from our little donor Angel, forever grateful—- and he is now living his best life. Organ donation does save lives. This changed me to my core.

I have developed a deep love of knowledge and expanded my mindset. Challenging and up-leveling any limiting beliefs; I don't want them to hold me back; I firmly believe in creating the energy of abundance. The world's communities consciously lack the abundance mindset; it's natural to step into that lack mentality. We aren't taught to increase our vibration of abundance and sit in that space. I focus on doing this for my family and within my work. The power to create the change in yourself, then everything changes around you. I integrate and expand my self-development daily alongside staying connected to my heart. I challenge you inspiring you to create your guide to wellness. What is going into your chosen energetic being for your travels forward in life? Because magnetic grace is my choice, and the option is yours. Find me at bossaesthetics.com.au, and on socials. My 'Glow Facial Club is my signature 12-month membership program for local QLD clients to invest in themselves, a bespoke anti-aging and scarring program treatment course.

I'd love to connect with you; reach out to me for a chat.

About the Author

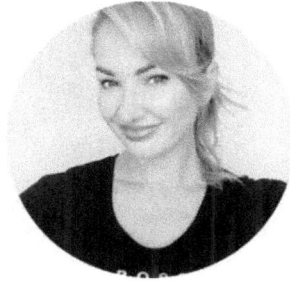

Fiona Louise Ireland, owner-operator of Boss Aesthetics. A career in the beauty industry spanning almost 30 years planted her solid roots were the beginnings of old-fashioned styled beauty therapy where you nurtured your client's skin & soul. Government Accredited Training in Paramedical and Cosmetic Tattoo Artistry and finalist in the ABATA (Australian Beauty and Cosmetic Tattoo Awards) for best 3D Areola Tattoo.

Melbourne-born, yet the sunrays were a magnet for living the dream sunshine-drenched- lifestyle close to the magnificent beaches of the Gold Coast QLD. Now living within walking distance of her favorite beach in Miami, Fiona is bringing up her two giant sizes in stature teenage sons, Kai & Levi. She has a gorgeous daughter Kiara who has happily flown the coup to spread her adult wings into her designed future.

Website: bossaesthetics.com.au
Email: bosaesthetics3@gmail.com
Instagram: @bossaesthetics_skin

-WW→

Tahlia Oliver

The beginning

I grew up in a relatively small town in the picturesque landscapes of Queensland, Australia, where our backyard was the world-famous Whitsundays (which includes the Great Barrier Reef). It was the kind of town where we never needed a map to find our way around. We knew all the streets and could find our way to our friend's house because we were familiar with the town. I have a lifetime of memories and friendships here from my childhood. I studied at University here and could have found a role and stayed my entire life in this town. However, a series of events that had recently taken place had a negative impact on my feeling about this town, my future, and my general well-being. In my final year of high school and before starting University, my family and I suffered two significant losses in the space of a few months.

The first blow struck when my beloved Grandfather, who was an integral part of my life, suddenly became ill with a cancerous brain tumor. In the space of as few as 3 months from his diagnosis, he had lost his battle with this brain cancer and passed away. As a result, I missed completing my final year of high school while coping with the grief of losing my grandfather. The absence of my grandfather, this integral figure in my life, left a void that seemed impossible to fill, and I grappled with grief. Life felt like a much more challenging and colder place without him around. He was such a vital support to me and my family in so many ways.

Within months of losing my grandfather, we suffered another loss. A natural disaster had struck our town leaving destruction in its wake. After hours and hours of torrential rains, our home was in an area susceptible to flooding, and we had about 4ft of water throughout our entire house. We lost everything, furniture, cars, belongings, and memories. The torrential floods washed away not just our physical possessions but also our sense of security and stability. Our entire house was destroyed and needed to be rebuilt, so we were left uncertain, moving around from home to home, losing the strength we once knew.

Following these events, I found my friendships strained because of my grief (and perhaps resentment that I had to experience this while others didn't), and I felt trapped in a rut. My feelings about the town I had grown up in and my outlook on life, in general, became shrouded with overwhelming negativity. I felt that life had become very stagnant, and if I did not make a significant change, I would not make much of my life and instead become quite self-destructive. It was a dark period in my life, but for some reason, I felt that I could achieve more and longed for a change.

Once I had finished my University degree, I decided to apply for roles in the largest capital cities in Australia, which were a long way from my hometown. I decided I needed to challenge myself and change my environment to get out of this negative rut I felt I was in. I had applied to several leading global companies and impressed those interviewing me at a leading international firm at their Melbourne office in Australia. This role was the deciding factor that I needed to move away from my hometown and to a large city where I knew no one over a 3-hour flight from my hometown.

Initially, I didn't realize the transformational impact this would have on my life and how this would contribute toward positive mental and physical health. It wasn't until about 6 years later, when I experienced another traumatic event that impacted my health and well-being that I realized the power of travel and moving to new places.

During my most recent traumatic experience, I received a lot of exposure to various psychiatric specialists, techniques, and practices. This included advice on meditative practices, occupational therapy, mindfulness, CBT, and others. I mainly learned that with many of these practices, I had to find a way to apply them so they would be effective for me. I realized traveling was one of the ways I had effectively applied a number of these practices, how it was healing for me, and how it allowed me to transform my life for the better.

Transformation Journey

Traveling has been an incredible journey of self-discovery and personal growth for me. It has provided a transformative experience that has helped me address various life challenges, heal, and grow to be the best version of myself. I have found traveling a powerful tool, which has formed one of my rules for wellness as it has helped me in the following ways:

- Recover from Trauma
- Practice Mindfulness and Gratitude
- Meditative Practices and Sensory Relief
- Challenging me to Grow
- Renew and Invigorate my Life
- Support Networks and Friendships

Recover from Trauma - One of the key benefits I have discovered is that traveling allows me to heal from trauma by creating a safe space to feel secure enough to address the pain and move forward. Leading studies on those impacted by trauma and suffering from PTSD have shown that people cannot heal from trauma while they still feel like they are in an unsafe environment. People must often be removed from an environment or a situation to feel safe enough to heal. This was a very relatable situation for me, and I found myself staying in the same place I felt unable to move on from the negative feelings I had. When I travel to new places, I think I can distance myself from the triggers and stressors of my traumatic experiences, creating a sense of safety and security. This safe environment has provided me the space to heal from trauma, process this event and emotions, and begin healing.

Practice Mindfulness and Gratitude - Another key mindfulness practice I have achieved through traveling is gratitude and appreciation.

Through my travels, I have been to countries where the majority of society ranges from some of the highest income per capita in the world to countries where most of the population lives under the poverty line. Both of these ends of the spectrum have given me gratitude and appreciation for the world we live in. Seeing some of the most innovative societies where people live so comfortably and have beautiful homes and beautiful gardens has made me appreciate how beautiful life can be. But equally, I have experienced beauty in some of the most remote places where nature is incredible. Still, the people genuinely have little by way of material possessions and financial wealth. Seeing how people can find happiness in some of the simplest things, like going for a swim together with their friends on the beach in the afternoon, even though they all are living below the poverty line, has really helped me put things into perspective and learn to enjoy the moment.

I can also reflect on the many photos I have taken during my travels, particularly during challenging times, and appreciate the amazing things I have been able to see and experience in my life. I can stop and think how beautiful and diverse our world truly is.

Practicing gratitude can help change our mindset from focusing on the negative of the now to appreciating the blessings we have had in life.

Traveling and seeing different perspectives has helped me to practice gratitude.

Meditative Practices and Sensory Relief - Exposure to Occupational Therapy and Cognitive Behavioral Therapy to support with psychological distress I was experiencing during a traumatic event has given me insights into tools I can utilize to ensure my mental well-being.

Through Occupational Therapy, I have learned to understand positive and negative sensory triggers and how this can help mitigate anxiety or adverse reactions to situations.

Through Cognitive Behavioral Therapy, I have learned the importance of not getting caught in negative thinking patterns and finding ways to stop reoccurring negative thoughts. Traveling is a way I can effectively apply both techniques.

When traveling, my mind is stimulated by the positive sensorial factors around me—for example, the beautiful sights and smells of walking through flower gardens and smelling fresh flowers. Or walking through a traditional old souk (market) in the Middle East and smelling the oud (fragrances) burning. Hearing the incredible music sung in local languages, I do not understand—experiencing beautiful nature sceneries or feeling the cold crisp air on my face when it is -10 degrees outside in Lapland in Finland. These and other sensory factors have a calming effect on me and help me stay relaxed, particularly in stressful situations.

Also, the mental challenge and learning mindset I am in when I am somewhere new, seeing something I have never seen before, or traveling to a destination I have never been to is something I find effective in keeping my mind busy. I do not engage in ongoing negative thinking patterns when my mind is active. I am distracted by the learning and challenge of being somewhere new and the sense of achievement when I leave a new country after traveling there alone successfully. This change in the way I am thinking is almost meditative for me. Paired with this, I get considerable physical exercise when walking, hiking, or exploring new locations. This physical exercise is something I don't even find a chore/burden when traveling and provides an obvious benefit to my mental health and overall well-being.

Renew and Reinvigorate my life - I have also found that traveling or relocating has allowed me to "renew" or "reinvigorate" my life.

Traveling or relocating to a new place, particularly alone, allows you to redefine yourself and let go of the past. If you travel somewhere nobody knows you from the past, your successes or failures do not define you. People do not know your history, and you can choose how much to share and when you choose to share this. I have found that when I have traveled and relocated, I can start "fresh" as the best version of myself. The person I have grown to become today is the person that people are seeing. It becomes an opportunity to level up into who you want to be in life and continue striving to be your best version. You don't become defined by your past failures or who you used to be. I feel if I would not travel and if I stayed in my hometown, I would have been constrained to act the way that people considered to be authentic to me and to not "change" too much. Moving and traveling have allowed me to evolve and constantly challenge myself to be the best version of myself and who I genuinely want to be.

Challenging me to Grow - It has also opened my horizons to learning new things, challenging my perspectives, and stepping out of my comfort zone. Embracing different cultures and customs has helped me confront my biases and preconceived notions. It has expanded my horizons and encouraged a more open-minded and adaptable approach to life. My challenges and obstacles during my travels have allowed me to develop problem-solving skills, resilience, and resourcefulness. Each new experience has been an opportunity for personal growth, as I have learned to navigate uncharted territories and embrace the unknown. These experiences have shaped me into a more confident and adaptable individual.

Support Networks and Friendships - Besides appreciating the world, traveling has allowed me to realize the inherent goodness in people and build new relationships. Sometimes, the people closest to us may inadvertently contribute to our challenges or hold us back from personal growth. Sometimes the people we feel are closest to us are only closest to us because of our physical proximity (such as dealing with them daily at work or because they live close to us). They may be holding us back or not the best people to have in our lives. By venturing into unfamiliar territories and interacting with individuals from diverse backgrounds, I have been amazed by the kindness, generosity, and warmth that exist in people across the globe.

These encounters have shattered stereotypes and reaffirmed my belief in the goodness of humanity.

Building new relationships while traveling has been a significant source of personal growth and support. The connections I have formed along my travels have broadened my perspective, exposed me to different cultures, and enriched my understanding of the world. These meaningful connections have provided me lifelong friendships, positive influences, and a sense of belonging that transcends geographical boundaries. I have established a friendship network and source of support that exists globally. I have also now found myself in the happiest, most loving, safe relationship I have experienced. This would never have occurred if I had not sought to change my environment and travel.

The Future

In conclusion, the benefits of traveling have been immeasurable in my life. It has provided a safe space for healing from trauma. It has allowed me to cultivate gratitude and appreciation for the world. Travel has facilitated the realization of the goodness in people and the formation of new relationships. I have broadened my perspectives and established a great friendship circle. By creating the right environment around me, traveling has led to a greater level of happiness and contributed to my personal and professional success. It has been a transformative journey of self-discovery, growth, and healing that I will forever cherish.

I have established myself in my career, experiencing incredible growth and gaining recognition on a global scale for my capabilities and expertise. The new friendships and positive influences I have encountered through traveling have played a significant role in this success, as they have provided unwavering support to me. Travel is the reward I give myself after substantial achievements. It is the way I maintain my health in significant periods of stress. Most importantly, it is the way I have healed myself after substantial trauma.

Often when people see my pictures or hear my stories, I encourage them to at least once just experience traveling solo to a country they have never thought of going to, and I speak of the benefits I have found doing so. I share my photography and experiences on my travels to demonstrate the beauty in the world that can be found when you take an adventure. If traditional measures of meditation or well-being are not working for you, I recommend going on an adventure, as this may work for you just as it did for me.

About the Author

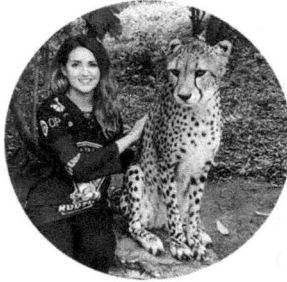

Tahlia was born in Australia to an Australian Mother and a Finnish Father. She graduated from University with a Bachelor of Information Technology in Australia.

She has vast experience working at leading global professional services firms and has worked across Australia, the United States, Asia, and the Middle East. She has published several well-received articles and thought leadership pieces in her field of expertise (Digital Transformation and Enterprise Agility).

Tahlia has a passion for traveling and tries to see at least 3 new countries every year (a goal she has easily broken year after year without fail). She loves to take travel photography on her trips to share the beauty she sees worldwide.

Email: Tahlia.Oliver@hotmail.com
Instagram: @tahltahl
LinkedIn: linkedin.com/in/tahliaoliver

-ᨆᨆ→

Scott Raven

*"I've missed more than 9,000 shots in my career. I've lost
almost 300 games. Twenty-six times I've been trusted to take
the game-winning shot and miss. I've failed over and over and
over again in my life. And that is why I succeed."* – Michael
Jordan.

The True Pursuit of Wealth and Well-Being

For many years, I was raised and acted under the belief that the
growth of financial wealth was the most critical aspect of a well-
lived life. When I turned 40, I lived that exact definition of a
dream. I spent that day at the ballpark with my work team as
part of a team outing and later had a wonderful dinner with my
family where my son lost not one, but two of his baby teeth. I
was living the definition of a well-lived life grounded in
pursuing financial wealth. Little did I know then how misguided

I was and all I have learned since. And it is through all that I've learned since that drives my purpose – to aid those seeking a valid combination of wealth and well-being through their professional pursuits to achieve the lives they desire.

In 2017, when I lost my executive position, which had become a large part of my identity, I fell into a severe depression that led to poor health decisions. Those decisions came to a head just before Christmas. I picked the kids up from school and felt severe pains in my chest, head, and back. As we returned to the house and were about to sit down for dinner, I pulled my wife aside and said I needed to go to the ER. In the ER, they immediately pulled me into the back room and took my blood pressure reading.

It was 180/110.

A battery of tests would follow to ensure there wasn't something immediately fatal in my system. Fortunately for me and my family, there wasn't. It did not turn out to be a heart attack or any other severely debilitating condition– just severe hypertension. I had fallen victim, by default, to my health trade-offs and ended up sacrificing my health, specifically in the form of depression and anxiety-induced alcoholism. As I lay there in the ER bed, being prepped to be admitted into the hospital for overnight observation, my family could come back and visit me. My son, who was seven then, could only know I wasn't feeling well and wanted to ensure I was OK. I was trying to think if that was the last moment I spent with him and what I wanted him to hear from me. That alone is a harrowing thought indeed. One that I don't wish upon anyone. That event started my evolving and never-ending journey of self-awareness and self-discovery.

I was trying to understand exactly who I was after I had been laid off from my executive-level role. That role defined a large part of my identity then; I had no sense of self without it. I was financially well off between what my wife and I had saved plus the severance coming in, so I knew I had time concerning money. And I wasn't in any mood to burden those around me with the myriad of negative self-talk going through my head, so I made it a point not to burn any relationships I had due to my struggles. Over the next six months, I would learn mindsets, lifestyle changes, medicines, and techniques that would allow me to keep my blood pressure under relative control. I vowed I would never make trade-offs for my health again.

Fast forward to the end of 2019.

I was in a transition period. After re-entering the workforce, my position was eliminated as part of a multi-billion-dollar merger. I had a disdain for corporate America and didn't want to put myself in a place where I relied on corporate America for my health. I decided I was going to move on from corporate America.

At that time, my son was having fun in martial arts, and an opportunity presented itself for me to start a business in the space. The universe was sending me signals that this was my next move, and because all that was required at first was the initial investment, I didn't have to worry about the realized financial implications for a bit. But I knew I was still in a period where not everything was clear—the nebulousness of the situation did not sit well with me.

Unlike in 2017, I knew I could not let my thoughts simply fester in my head. So by default, I ended up burdening my friends with my emotions. I needed them to help keep me calm during this period of transition. And one by one, several of them put up the sign—some implicitly by checking out, others more directly—that I had violated their boundaries. Many are now lost from my life. The damage had been done and didn't sit well with me. I vowed I would never allow myself to lose meaningful relationships in that manner again. The period immediately after I entered the martial arts space was fun. It was NOT corporate America, and anything different from where I came from was good. But you can only run away from things for so long without running toward something meant for you. I consistently learned that lesson as the days, months, and years passed.

Towards the end of 2021, the learning pains associated with operating the new business venture, along with unforeseen circumstances, such as the prolonged impact of COVID, were taking its toll. The business needed to be fixed the way I had projected, far from it, and I knew I needed to address it. This was for my sake and my primary stakeholders— my wife and family and the employees whose livelihood depended on me. It was a charge I took very seriously. I had developed enough mental fortitude that while it was a stressful situation, it wasn't nebulous. I was determined to see things through, so I wasn't experiencing poor health. And I had learned my lessons from two years ago... this was my mess to own, and I was going to take ownership without overly burdening others. So by default, I spent a necessary resource to turn things around— wealth. The business needed me to inject more of my time, money, and focus into it for it to turn around.

I also set limits on how much longer I would give myself on this venture and asked my wife to hold me accountable. I knew I would be emotionally charged to continue so as "not to fail." When the time came, and with the significant help of my wife, who held me to my promise to her and the family, I exited the business. And I did so without regrets— I had given it my all and could walk away from its sunk costs.

When I got far enough past the event to review it, I realized I had invested in something that needed to be in my zone of genius, and it was a venture that I was running towards. It needed to be truly aligned with my purpose and passion. I vowed that if I ever retook an entrepreneurial risk, I would apply these lessons regarding wealth and alignment. After all that I had been through, I needed to hit the pause button before jumping back into professional life.

There was self-discovery, self-awareness, and self-reflection work to be done.

There were statements of forgiveness and gratitude that needed to be said.

There were parts of my life that were over.

These were necessary seasons of my life, and I'm glad they occurred. As the great Vin Scully said, "Don't be sad because it's over." Plus, I had two important anchors in my life.

In the same period since I was 40, all of these necessary live events were happening for me. My family and marathon running were also constant sources of strength. My charitable marathon running began through my sister as she convinced me to join the team one year after she did, raising money to see the end of cancer in memory of our late Mom and focusing on pursuing goals larger than myself.

One way that manifested itself is through a young boy from New Hampshire, Max, who I had the privilege of running on behalf of in 2018 as his patient partner. No five-year-old should ever have to face cancer, particularly not one so full of life as Max. And his smiling face and disposition on life were one of the main things that drove me that year in what many have called "The Run Through The Washing Machine" – steady rain, 30 mph headwinds, and cold temps made it one of the most memorable Marathon Mondays on record. Many abandoned the race, but I did not because of Max. So when Max's parents announced that his cancer had returned in 2022, it was straightforward for me to want to run for him again.

As I began my marathon training and fundraising efforts, I was learning how much doing so positively impacted every part of me.

Every tough mile, every reach out for donations and support – all of them were challenges I faced with a smile because I knew what I wanted to provide Max and all those afflicted with cancer because of my efforts. In short, I now had found my true definition of a life filled with wealth and well-being. More importantly, I was prepared to take the steps necessary to manifest my purpose through my actions.

As I write this, I see how much I've changed and grown. And I see clearly how the recent events in my life, and all the wisdom it has provided me, allowed me to launch my coaching practice with peace and perspective. My efforts are aligned with my passion and purpose, and I'm running towards this opportunity with authentic engagement because it helps fuel my soul.

I realized that the reasons I live the life I do were the same as when I went into the martial arts space in 2019 – but unlike then, when the purpose was to run away from my past, I now know what I'm running towards.

My coaching practice is grounded on helping aspiring entrepreneurs achieve the wealth and well-being they desire while fulfilling their purpose, aligned with their core values.

My decisions are grounded in taking a calculated entrepreneurial risk and considering the potential impact on my primary stakeholders -- my wife and family.

My tribe of like-minded individuals who genuinely want to see me and all of us succeed grows by the day, allowing me to have both quantity and quality support to guide me.

And my focus on my health is now innate -- I don't even have to think about it. I just do it because it's an essential element of my identity. All these lessons are now wisdom I can happily share with others to give them the gifts I have been blessed enough to receive – to pay forward what I've learned to improve others.

If you've made it this far, thank you for allowing me to share my story.

I would love to know the reasons why my story resonated with you.

You may feel stuck and unhappy in your current profession and long for something more aligned with your soul. Perhaps you are fearful and scared of leaping. – what if something goes wrong? What if I'm not successful?

I want to remind you of the quote Teddy Roosevelt delivered known as "The Man in the Arena":

"It is not the critic who counts, not the man who points out how the strong man stumbles or where the doer of deeds could have done them better. The credit belongs to the man who is actually in the arena, whose face is marred by dust and sweat and blood; who strives valiantly; who errs, who comes short again and again, because there is no effort without error and shortcoming; but who does strive to do the deeds; who knows great enthusiasms, the great devotions; who spends himself in a worthy cause; who at best knows, in the end, the triumph of high achievement, and who at the worst, if he fails, at least fails while daring greatly, so that his place shall never be with those cold and timid souls who neither knows victory nor defeat."

You are beautiful. You are strong. You are meant for great things. And if you are willing to bet on yourself and dare to be great, you will be blessed with the powerful experiences that come with it. If you're ready to leap yourself or even just chat about beliefs and thoughts that have spurred within you because of listening to my story, I'm here to listen to you.

I have been blessed to have all these experiences to realize my true self-worth by learning to be loyal to myself.

My calling is to help others experience the success, pride, satisfaction, and fulfillment of passionately pursuing their purpose through their professional endeavors.

I know my composition is meant to allow people to be vulnerable – to share their fears, self-doubts, and limiting beliefs – so that they can be addressed and not let them be barriers to the life of wealth and well-being they genuinely wish to pursue.

Become the version of yourself that you genuinely wish to be.

"We delight in the beauty of the butterfly but rarely admit the changes it has gone through to achieve that beauty" -- Maya Angelou.

And that I'm here to help you because I've been there. You can too.

As I look back in summary throughout my journey, it hasn't been one for the faint of heart.

It's had me looking into my son's eyes, wondering if I would see him again the next day.

It's been one which started a series of positive and negative events that have shaped me into the person I am today.

It's been one which has seen me lose money, good friends, and the charisma of what my life was supposed to be.

But...

It has also opened my eyes to all the lessons I needed to learn, particularly about myself. It has taught me about things that are indeed inside of me -- perseverance, resilience, and yes, self-loyalty and loyalty of those around me -- that I didn't know existed in me at such levels.

It has provided me with many scars, but I wear them proudly and use them as fuel for what I want going forward, not as a crutch to be a victim forever.

While the outcomes along the way have been painful at times, I embrace the experience that came with it and the core part of the message it allows me to share with others.

I hope my message and call to action serve you well.

Thank you for taking the time for me to share my story with you, and I wish you nothing but the best as you pursue your dreams of wealth and well-being.

- Scott

About the Author

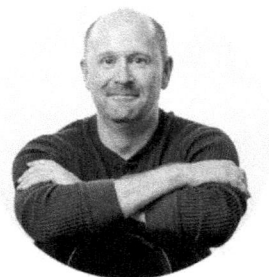

Scott Raven is an empowerment and entrepreneurial coach focusing on aspiring and recent entrepreneurs. His mission is to help accomplished professionals live their purpose and find a balance of wealth and well-being. He has a Bachelor's degree in computer science from the University of Pennsylvania and an MBA from the Tepper School of Business at Carnegie Mellon University.

He's also opened two martial arts studios in the Atlanta area, allowing students to experience personal physical improvement as well as mental and emotional growth. A seven-time marathon runner for charity on behalf of the Dana-Farber Cancer Institute, he has raised over $125,000 for innovative basic cancer research.

He lives in Atlanta with his wife Kham and their two children, and loves getting together with close friends for coffee, or beers, and spending time with his kids,

LinkedIn: www.linkedin.com/in/scott-raven
Email: contact@scottraven.com

-ww→

Candace Reed

Let's go on Rainbow Safari.

There is no desire that anyone holds for any other reason than to believe they will feel better in achieving it. Whether it is a material object, a physical state of being, a relationship, a condition, or a circumstance."At the heart of every desire is the desire to feel good " –Esther Hicks. A rainbow will appear in the sky when you least expect it; hope, inspiration, acceptance, beauty after the storm, and all-embracing love— A journey of one's natural habitat. As we navigate through life and experience the vibrancy from a perspective of color and harbor the outlook and intention of living with ambition for a sizeable well-lived life, we will be complete.

I've dived deep over the years into dark realms and ended up as stagnant many times. No stranger to hard work or a challenge, I have overcome and felt more robust each time. Over time I discovered the magic of alignment, energy, and intention. Allowing connection. Always pondering...Is there more— is there another spectrum we can exist — a prism of life, a way of looking and thinking? The law of attraction, if you will—your thoughts powering your ability to change the world. If you are unhappy—growth is absent, and your world is not full of Rainbows. Yet, change will set your intention to move forward— gracefully, with Gusto!

Rainbow Safari

I AM. I am many things. I am complex. I am energetic. I am busy and desire a natural result for my efforts. I AM a Chameleon, constantly changing to suit my environment.

I AM. I am excited about the future, for new realms and new journeys. I am currently in the creation and dreaming phase, combining my many passions to develop a way to share a wholesome, holistic, and adventurous experience with my clients.

I have come to realize along my life's Safari that it's the little things that are the most important and valuable. These are the lessons taught to us by our Elders, Friends, and Family, and those who cross our path. These lessons taught me to wake up daily and accept a new deep gratitude. Our minds are fantastic assets; I enjoy diving deep into mine to reach knowledge and direct experience—there have been many, both incredible and wonderful and joyous, and some not so much. With darkness comes light, and it's not wise to wander around in the dark where there are potentially harmful things for too long without remembering your own inner light. Our vast minds are like Outerspace, often filled with floating junk and exploding stars. My philosophy has been to not live in your past pain, experiences, and questionable life choices. We have our memories and our darker experiences—these are often what shape us. We do not need to unpack and live there. Pack a new bag, or just leave the bag behind and start fresh. MOVE!

"HAPPY BIRTHDAY," read the sign.

The Bell Tent we just finished setting up will undoubtedly be received later in the day with squeals of delight and wonder— SUPRISE!

A birthday girl was experiencing the joy of sharing a sleepover with friends— Magical memory-making moments. She is transported to Rainbow Safari. Entering the multicolored tent, visions of bright colors mix with animal print rugs, cushions, and decor, creating a place for connection and magic.

My vision is again changing and aligning with my new goals, values, and intentions. Combining my previous Ayurveda knowledge, Massage Therapy, Energy Healing experience, Spa treatments, and Holistic Herbal knowledge with our Best

Intentions Tent and Events Company— My colorful imagination is my Oyster. The Pearl: my far-reaching passion and desire for more.

The Best InTenTions Tent Co. is our Event Planning business— Bell Tent Villages for events, Festivals, and Weddings. Children's Parties, Outdoor Cinemas, picnics, and so much more. A fulfilling and incredible journey of connection, laughter, and memories.

Our planet is slowly returning to in-person gatherings, and we, too, want more of this—More connection, growth, healing, and conversation. We as humans must come together in a community and gather. Dance, Laugh, Talk, and Breathe.

What am I doing? I AM growing the seeds, fertilizing the gardens of my mind. I am still determining my future direction precisely, and I am OK with that as long as it involves growth. I have an exceptionally supportive partner who is all in. All in for the clarity, the distortion, the geometry, and the bending of the light—Just like the facets of a Rainbow.

If I could tell my younger self anything, it would be to learn to rest more. Relax, Revive, Renew. I'm a Go-Go-Go person who never stops until I drop. I have been on a 5-year cycle of building myself up, changing my passions, work, and businesses, and then feeling like I need to move and grow, plant new seeds. Up and down all my life, people close to me tragically left this earth too early. Year after year in my younger life and then too often in my later years. At many of these points, there was nothing to bring me back except breath and feeding my brain with more knowledge to bring myself forth from these darker moments.

I LOVE LIFE— learning, exploration and travel, self-expansion, interest in other people's journeys, energy connection, and movement. It often leaves me feeling upset and confused to see others with the fear of not wanting to be better, the fear of change—Metathesiophobia. How can it be? Those who are afraid of changing and growing to their full potential, I don't fully understand. I see the challenges; I have felt them, too, repeatedly. But, I have questions, curiosity, and wanting more. A desire to be stronger, more knowledgeable, MORE!

I often find myself enquiring about what is happening in my life. What was I doing?I just don't know this! I was consistent here, though. I don't wallow; I try not to complain or moan. I've changed it.

A catalyst for me was when I was 23. I found myself in darkness, wearing black (this hasn't changed I still love wearing black!), and making choices that were not on a path of Sunshine and Rainbows. I became more potent when I decided I would not be living unhappily and in this state of grief and loss. Behind each smile was an intense sadness that no one could see or feel. That was enough. I actively went out of my way to cognitively awake and make my own choices. Now I deal with whatever comes my way with strength and as a wiser person. Each day I choose Life, Gratitude, Honesty, and Learning.

A significant highlight was diving into the Ocean's depths so peacefully away from the business of terra-firma-life, descending below the turbulent surface and hearing nothing but my breath, heartbeat, and the Scuba tank bubbling. Nothing— only enjoyment on the diving guests' faces and the unfolding colors of the coral reefs, the fish, our Turtle community— 'Turtley awesome' underwater friends. Facilitating Scuba Diving Boat Tours was one of those 'past things' I used to do. I loved feeling the weightlessness and buoyancy and experiencing what covers over 70% of the earth's surface. Ocean life is magical; it's a whole different world. I know I have not been diving for five years now, yet I continue paying my license fees and will return to it. Cyclone Debbie ripped through Mackay in March 2017, stopping everything. It was a category four system, and our whole world changed. Then, not too long after, the world locked down due to 'pandemica', and most businesses were on their ears, glad things had changed. It is funny how we experience chaos and disaster during storms and catastrophes, yet, out of it, we again rise to a sense of clarity....Time for something new. A Rainbow!

Eat the Rainbow

"I can't eat anymore stinking Pizza. I don't understand"! I found myself saying.

I arrived at gut, joint, physical, and mental health. Breathe, Eat, Move, and Mantras are my cheat code to life, more like a THRIVE code.

Why not encode and begin to find the answers for myself? My life, body, and health are changing, and I set out to discover the answers to what was happening. In turn, I found so much knowledge and information I couldn't get enough of each new idea, and the science, love it all —- to assist myself and others and ditch the Stinkin' Pizza! I liked it, but it didn't like me.

With all my traveling and experiencing life, I moved back to Mackay to assist my Mother in her Spa and returned to the wellness and Beauty industry. Mum had built a new clinic with a fantastic Spa and float tank space–Natural Body and Beauty Clinic Day Spa. I now had a space for my Ayurveda massage, and we have an extraordinary Australina-made botanical range which I LOVE! My zest for all things WHOLE ignited. I want to express the natural magic, nutrition, and enlightenment behind self-care, self-nurturing, and DEEP REST. I liked this for me, I wanted to provide this as a practitioner, and I wanted this for my clients—the healing nature of sound, vibration, breathing, movement, and botanicals. I personalize the therapies to align with what the clients are currently experiencing.

I seek to personalize our offering of therapies and spa rituals. I often play healing journey music if they need elevating or specially selected oils and massage strokes to evoke intense healing, deep emotional release, and freedom.

"The Deep relaxation and botanicals transported me to another place," stated a recent client after her Spa treatment with us—a self-care-indulgence-spa experience, traversing their lives, stresses, and chaos. My future vision is expanding far beyond and applying my skills and knowledge to a retreat in nature - how blissful. Will it happen? I'm not sure. Indeed, my image is fantastic, and I would even book in for that as a client.

We also possess some unique books in our clinic space that have changed my life, and when purchased by our clients, I hear of the protocols they have followed—-life-changing experiences are the result, and their gut health, skin, and the inner world have changed too.

One of these books is 'Gut Skin Connections' by Janine Tait (Janine Tait Group Ltd, 2019), a New Zealand-based Naturopath. The book had been designed for the skin and beauty clinics to assist in helping our clients to achieve the skin of their dream. We have this reality available for sale at all times.

One Recipe that has changed my life entirely is the Sweet carrot and apple recipe.

'Gut Skin Connections' by Janine Tait,(Janine Tait Group Ltd, 2019, p 36)

EXERT:

"THE GUT-SKIN CONNECTION" publication is 224 full-color pages book by author Janine Tait, combining new advances in gut research with holistic skincare wisdom, providing the principles, recipes, rituals, and a meal plan to restore your gut and renew your skin from within.

THE RESEARCH IS CLEAR. IF YOU WANT TO TRANSFORM YOUR SKIN, YOU NEED TO LEARN HOW TO LOVE AND CARE FOR YOUR GUT.

All the recipes are gluten-free, dairy-free, and refined sugar-free.

Sweet Carrot and Apple recipe:

INGREDIENTS

Two servings
1 carrot, peeled and grated
1 apple, cored and grated
Juice of 1/2 a lemon

2 tablespoons of coconut thread

1 tablespoon of raisins or sultanas

2 teaspoons of olive oil

1 teaspoon of raw honey

½ a teaspoon of ground cinnamon

½ a teaspoon of ground ginger

TO SERVE

1 tablespoon of coconut yogurt (dairy free)

1 tablespoon of Bestow Beauty Plus Oil

Suitable for: Breakfast

METHOD

Mix all ingredients except olive oil in a bowl and mix well—heat olive oil in a large frypan for a couple of minutes at med-high heat. Add the mixed ingredients and sauté until soft and fragrant (5 – 10 minutes).

PROGRAMME NOTES

Serve half warm with yoghurt and Bestow Beauty Plus Oil. Place the other half in a sealed container in the fridge for breakfast on Day 2. We put ours in a glass jar along with the yoghurt and Bestow Beauty Plus Oil so that we can easily take a portable breakfast to work if we wish to.

NOTES: This is one of our favorite breakfasts, as it is equally delicious, served warm immediately or eaten cold the next day.

Simply use a carrot as the base and add fresh fruit (banana works nicely as it caramelizes), dried fruit, and spices. It tastes like a dessert and is a sweet treat you can enjoy that isn't detrimental to your gut health!

Rainbow Medicine

Healing through mother nature is wisdom. Herbal Medicine has inspired me to access more ancient knowledge, go back to what I already innately know, work what it and expand my experiences and skills. A coming back to self, again. The topical medicines, the internal medication, the nutritional therapies, and I am fascinated with all things Menopause and Female hormones– I would love to specialize in this area. I am experiencing hot flashes and have been told of peri-menopause effects on my body. The stress responses and the use of Ashwagandha, Saw Palmetto, and the simple garden variety Marjoram—the direct relation to hormones - to - Gut health is so interesting. Fascinating! Life changing!

INSTEAD OF WEIGHT GAIN—-HEALTHY CHANGE.

INSTEAD OF DIGESTION ISSUES—A BALANCE.

INSTEAD OF HOT FLASHES—ENTER THE HERBS AND TEAS WHICH HELPED THEM.

As a child, my favorite activity was looking for Fairies, rock hopping, searching for waterfalls, and going out in nature. I lived both in town and out of town with two parents. As an adult, it's not a surprise that I tap into my inner child. I am very fond of the outdoors, nature, and energy—I still like spending time with Fairies! This is a level of self-care for me— make time for yourself! I love a good tea as medicine; this one is my favorite:

Detox tea recipe: Homemade Detox Tea: Lemon, Ginger, and turmeric.

This tea is my go-to, a way to start the day and the best way to end a hectic weekend.

When I say "detox," I do not mean cleanse or meal replacement, but immune support and healthy digestion tea.

INGREDIENTS AND METHOD: Hot water, Lemons—fresh slices and ½ lemon juice, Ginger–a chunk, Tumeric–a lump or the ground spice, Cinnamon stick, Cayenne pepper (optional). Combine the water, fresh Ginger and Lemon slices in a saucepan on a hot stove and boil. After 10 minutes, add Tumeric, Cayenne, and Cinnamon stick (or ground Cinnamon) and simmer for another 10 minutes. Remove from heat and stand to cool. Add the ½ lemon juice. Use it as a concentration or a shot if you desire.

Breathe the Rainbow

"I love you, thank you, respect you, and protect you," I repeat as my daily mantra while breathing into my belly. Silences my brain and heads into a place of rest.

Pilates, Yoga, Cold-Water Plunges, and Music have all driven my transformational journey. Certain Megahertz drive away certain aggravating factors. A simple combination of Pilates and Massage, "Can I do this once a month?" Spa clients ask me. I explain how releasing the trapped energy, addressing their feelings, the healing power of a touch, healing sounds, and aromatics are medicinally beneficial. "Why not twice a month?" Self-care is exfoliating the CR*P from your life that doesn't serve you. Honoring myself has made my journey all the difference. Intentionally changing my breathing pattern, releasing the mental clutter and the physical fatigue from the construction of the Tents, and my spiritual well-being is remembered in our busy days.

Incredible memories were looking for fairies. Such an idyllic sensory journey. Why not look for them now? KEEP IT SIMPLE - AND JUST FRIGGIN' BREATHE.

Best Intentions

Stop playing in the shadows and do the work. This was my

intention for the Best Intentions. Be open. Open to new beginnings, and be willing to alter the trajectory. There are so many closed-off, stale, and negative vibes in the world; don't render yourself in a state of toxicity to absorb it all.

My New Rule of Wellness is to wake up and makes sense of it all.

Let's honor each other, communicate better with the self, and have some self-honesty.

It's about choice, change, and intentions. My whole life has been a story of walking down the pathways of life with purpose; all the differences are I've done lots of walking and, in turn, lots of stepping out and walking away. That is my authentic truth. I love doing new things. I'm a different breed with a desire for 'something else.' I'm winning with the productivity demons, I'm winning with the pessimists, I'm winning with the detractors, and I'm winning within my little quirks of not liking being stagnant or stuck.

If you hate it, don't do it. If you hate it THAT MUCH, don't CONTINUE to do it.

The combination of all visible colors stems from a beam of light hitting the water or a prism; the light bends it depending on which way you are looking. From which perspective or spectrum do you look at your own life, experience your life and wake up to self-honesty? Within the energy of your quirks and individuality, it's up to you to step up, stay fresh or be an emotional doomsayer. Take a moment to immerse yourself in the world's natural beauty. Change it up and trust the process. Live every day a little more special than the last; it's up to you. It's the little things.

Contact me or pop into 10 Palmer Street, North Mackay–Aesthetics and Wellness at Natural Body Beauty Clinic.

About the Author

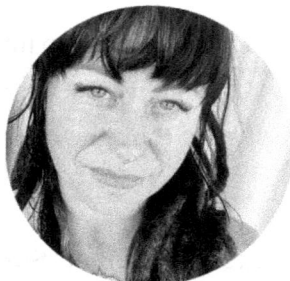

Candance Reed embraces the As-Above-So-Below principles; an exploration of our inner and outside worlds. Always choosing to grow, learn, and assist others to do the same through play, education, health, and joy. Currently, a celebrated Beauty and Skin/body Wellness Therapist and Day Spa/Skin Clinic Leader, working alongside her mother and a motivated team. Building her Glamping and Events business; creating spaces of joy and community; learning and building her expertise via studying Herbal Medicine, Pilates Teacher Training, and being a Breathwork facilitator.

Her world is her backyard garden—fab food and herbarium, her incredible partner Rowan, and fur-baby Basil. Exploring the amazing Australian Whitsunday region - Camping, Paddleboarding, collecting shells, and experiences. From Rum Bars to dusty dance floors; white beaches and turquoise waters, to backyard gardens and harmonious clinical spaces, there she is!

Website: www.bestintentionstentco.com
Website: www.naturalbodyandbeautyclinic.com.au
Facebook: https://facebook.com/thebestintentionstentco

-‏vvv→

Aiesha Rowles-Oliver

In the darkness, be the light.

Some of the best times of your life haven't happened yet; some have occurred in another life.

Our essence comes from the stars and will return at some stage; the In-between is up to you.

I found the spirit I longed for when in need of it and not a minute before. I adopted the art of learning and seeking. Songs, dance, frequency, and prayers honor the spirits of the land that I feel akin to. My heart's responding to the future. Within the understanding of soul direction and purification, allowing also occurs. Every thought and action we take can serve us well or add to our demise, and I am no different. I highlight that I've been through both, needing help understanding everything.

I sit here on the OTHER side of trouble, the healthy side of old concerns. I open my books and laptop, log in to my Holistic Nutrition and Herbal Medicine Course, and study. I have actively carved out time after putting the babies to bed for sleep. I feel like I am thriving, researching, studying, and writing—filling my cup; yet sometimes, I feel like I'm falling apart and living in chaos.

As I read about botanicals, nutritional science, herbal medicine, and health behavior, I channel my rebirth, seeing visions of ancient peoples under large trees and standing there with them. I look up from the thick trunk above the old knarled branches, a dew drop falling on my nose. One large bough dropped its twigs, and the fragrant evergreen aromas of the needle-like-leaves made their way to my nostrils; I felt the exposed root and mushrooms under my bare toes, and - I felt a connection to my origins, beginnings, the past, and now the future. Bringing my attention back to my study, I learned about herbal apothecaries and making tea and tinctures from this Cedar tree, 'The Tree of Life.' The same tree I saw in my vision. Like in a movie reel, I see myself sitting with other women, young and old, collectively, placing Cedar Springs in a pot, along with Rosemary, Thyme, and a Snow Fungus, swaying to the beat of drums. We add water and bring it to a boil. How do I know this is the ancient tribal remedy for Digestion, Vitaly, Hormone function, Liver, and Immunity? Because I've lived it—in another life.

I am in the right place in this life now.

I love sitting in the sunrays, eating foods that make me feel good. I love happiness—seeing others happy and a passion for herbal medicines. I use a Singing bowl in our lounge room when I feel frustrated or nearly going to pop. We play 528hz frequency music medicinally daily, and plenty of YouTube tunes belted out throughout our home to relax us all collectively. I chose *The World* card from my inspiration deck and invite myself to reflect on my journey and achievements and set goals for future fruition.

"Completion: Integration: Accomplishment: Journey Reflection. The World represents an end to a cycle of life, a pause. Stillness before the next cycle begins. An indicator of tectonic breadth"
(Biddy Tarot, Raide Waite cards, 2023.www.biddytarot.com)

Tectonic Beadth: big words >inexhorable change!

I know my life now is vastly changed from before— creating a family unit with my husband Mat and our two gorgeous kids, Indi and Koa; I don't know much about my childhood; I have a protection spell and a block in place for all my childhood memories. My sister sometimes tells me stories, and I do not recall that she is explaining another persona's life. I am often mood dependent, as is the house we live in. An excellent hand clap is the key to eradicating any stagnant energy. A good clap goes a long way.

My life changed when I had the children, and I changed when the kids were born. There is such a dogma around motherhood and parenting, no set rules, no handbook, and we become parents with a sparkle in our eyes. To then learn everyone has an opinion as to how we should raise our kids, what to feed them, how to treat them, what to educate them with, how to medicate them, "Why don't you come to do it yourself?" I feel like yelling at them!

My vision for impacting this world is to change this stigma somehow. It's so frustrating and becomes self-limiting. All I want is to not F*^CK up my kids, not to give them a crappy base to start their life, spiritually and holistically.

Our daughter has had a rough time entering this world this time around.

Mat had researched the 528 hz healing frequency, the 'love frequency,' and had played it ever since our daughter was in acute care. Essentially what the scan looked like, we were told, "holes in her brain," but we never stopped playing the music. Her health is still on and off; she is pale and can't eat at times, erratic and screams in pain, and passes out; it's an actual mind F*^CK to be fair, with no medical answers; it's a mystery.

A CORNER OF A BRICK WALL WOULD FEEL GOOD RIGHT ABOUT NOW!

A shower feels good to her, we often pop her under running water, and she loves the rain - hence her name—Indiana Rain. We wash away the bad energy, new start to feel good again, eradicate any lousy mood - wash away the negative energy, and I also do this as a soothing act as I did as a child. Indi screams— off to the shower we go; she stops immediately. Sometimes I run her foot under the tap water to use it as a calming tool and a diversion, allowing me to stop for a minute; it's heavenly.

Losses in my life have been aplenty, and not going into it all! Let's just say mental health has been a significant affliction in my close family, wider family, and friends; so many people sick and dying or have passed, and I often feel there is not even a stable person around me.

Having kids changed me entirely; adjusted myself to the core, and I feel like a different person, with positivity and hope. However, there is an existing FUNK; It's inside me, around me, in my mind. Let's normalize the funk; when I am IN the funk, I'm all off but feels natural. Everyone wants a way out, shows me the way, makes me better, fixes me, and has concerns for my welfare. I know I can do better even in the funk —is not wrong, it exists, and the funk I can't do much about. When I'm experiencing this—A thousand things are in my head, but simultaneously nothing at all—-all at once, over and over. It's so overwhelming, my head is on fire, and I can't put it down to particular things. There is a heavy cloud over me that I can't get out of, and I fight with my Ego, stamp my feet on the ground and clap my hands until I wake up out of my head for no apparent reason.

I was raised in a superstitious family and have adopted many traits, and mental health issues plagued us all. My Father tragically passed away by his hands, and I left Mum's house at 17.

One day at a friend's house, in a fairytale book, I read of a girl who couldn't see. She had enhanced senses, and this story resonated with me and stayed with me as an adult. It was set in the 1800s. These extra-sensory gifts this girl has mesmerized me, yet felt familiar.

Another book I read is also set in the 1800s time frame; a story about a girl who was to be hung for allegedly partaking in witchcraft, and towards the end of the story, was told people who sit with her, a priest, other people spoke to her and got to know her, the farmer got to know her—innocent, accused of all the wrong things and persecuted for her crimes that she didn't commit. They hanged her. I have extra-sensory perception, am Empathetic, and recall images and feeling from past existences, which had me guessing and thinking of persecutions and judgments of habits and quirks that still exist. Society is very judgey; people are opinionated and rude.

Darkness can not drive out darkness; only light can do that.

I always did things in even numbers; 2 drinks (which is still way out of control), drink water sips or gulps in even numbers> if it's not even, I spit it out, make sure a volume is an even number. Driving en route to a destination, I must go a long way around to double back on my route or come on a full circle- I will not go along a road that will go back on itself. Clothing too, left side, to right side, evenly. This is ruining everyone's life, others around me, and mine. It's ingrained in me that something terrible will happen if I don't do these things.

This OCD thing is controlling. I regularly Sage the house: white sage and Chant.

It's about me trying to get out of my head; when I do, my heart space is fantastic to live from. I want this for everyone, too, get out of your heads into your hearts more and open people up to see what the world has to offer—the beautiful world is there, even if everything is sucky in your life!

IN MY HEAD, I accept who we are, trying to jump on a timeline. I Relax a bit and enjoy more of life; living from the heart and healing energy is vital. Everyone takes extreme measures to deal with illnesses before the illness takes over.

Do better for yourself, and feel connected with your body; we are happier and less pressured to live in societal norms.

I have this reoccurring set of images—A dream? A vision? Still trying! But, It's a connection! I am wandering across a gorgeous open field with vast horizons and clear blue skies; I then become the land. I feel every creature's footstep, I feel every blade of grass moving on my surface, and I feel the breeze and sun rays fall across me. I AM. I am Mother Earth living and breathing, sustaining nature—watching, feeling, and providing for everything. As a human form again, I gulp water from a stream with my cupped hand, which feels like liquid magic; the cool sensation down the throat, I feel the clarity and refreshment, and I feel the connection to self. What a wonderful vision/dream/experience/meditation–whatever you want to call it. It's clarity to how I want to live right now-calmly, Total connection, total peace.

The next passion we support is Mat building a business with his brothers. I now have the opportunity to be at home nurturing our children and spending the delicious formative years with them; I know I am so blessed.

This is one of the reasons I am so passionate about Herbal Medicine and Inclusive Holistic Nutrition; healing my family from home and being tapped into ancient ways of medicine. Indi's health issues range from being purple, grey, and unconscious, looking malnourished, and having too many sensitivities to accelerating to behavioral. This has changed my view on health and highlighted that this is what I want to do with my life. Everyone struggles with various health issues, lifelong ailments, and inner turmoil.

The GAPS gut-mind-connection principle (Gut and Psychology Syndrome) has been life-changing for our family. By eliminating our pasteurized dairy, grains, starch, and refined carbohydrates, this diet has been instrumental for us. The imbalance of microbiome and mood correlation via evidence-based nutrition dietary protocol brings our results.

I am willing to release old, negative ways and beliefs. They are the only thoughts that stand in my way. My new thoughts are positive and fulfilling.

My nutritional platforms and information have been nearly impossible - searching for gut health but more natural ways. Information is available, but it's all similar to chemical-based supplementation, not readily available authentically natural solutions. We all want to live a better maximum. I've found the magic for Indi—Bone Broth stomach healer. The market is large, but I found a special Body Glue, and now I'm making our broth. We started a Special diet for Indi, and I gave her 1 teaspoon of natural bone broth glue in her bottles—- she wouldn't eat food, is a picky eater anyway, and has a loose bowl. Now eating heartily has formed stools and is all around a healthier little girl.

Her pale face has gone, completely changing her life and ours—
Gut lining health and far less inflammation.

I would love to see the distribution of nutritional information
more readily available. The study of Psychology of late includes
the survey around the gut-mind-link, and many health
professions are privvy; we need more information that Mums
and Dads can access to know more about the body connection
and understanding of body systems. So many parents are
Seeking for themselves alternate easy other than, "Take
panadol" or "Just eat vegetables," sometimes I just keep talking
and talking, and if feel nothing comes out of my mouth. I think
we're all sucked in, easy to get into, hard to get out of; it's all
troubling.

What would it be if you could take complete information to the
world?

At this point in my life, I feel that holistic herbal living, Nutrition,
and Spiritualism hold the space for finding my spiritual calling,
my higher self; still searching and learning, and figuring it all
out, what works and what doesn't work, a part of my higher self
wants me to be better, and do better for my family. This is my
higher self speaking. I want to promote the journey within it is
all-inclusive with nutrition.

My new rule of wellness is to embrace what you are passionate
about and remember to Dance. I haven't danced in years; move

my body, release. My wish, too, is for everyone to be seen as an equal—no shame, no lack, no one better than anyone else. Love and light for everyone.

To love is to see the light in everyone.

Being a mum is the most challenging job, even in personal adult relationships, and is an emotional rollercoaster. I only want to do better for them. I hate that everyone thinks they can have an opinion or the best advice on what to do and what not to do. Doing your best as a parent; loving them, taking time out, reading to them, crying along with them. " NO vegetables tight," "I can do better," let's understand we are all coping and managing, and let's be equal and show support. We need a whole village of mums; why am I a bad mum for relying on the town? Kids would come out and have a better chance at a good life if the mother wasn't always consumed with guilt.

Dealing with a teenager is a different application.

"I'll eat it later," and leaves it in the fridge to perish.

"Please don't read the ingredients," he says….. I read the label… and bin it.

I've Stopped buying things out of protest, yet I make a UP-AND-GO exception to keep the peace.

If I had all the time and money in the world, I'd want to take kids' places in nature, rainforests, and water holes down south. As they get older and travel to different countries, explore cultures, alternate ways of living and other foods, and share traditional tribal ways. I'm fortunate I don't have to return to work. I can stay with kids and experience their development, and we can spend all the time we need to nurture them. When you have a baby, every day brings new experiences. I have to say the 'shitty-nappies-syndrome' has befallen Mat; it is intrinsically like a plague. I feel like saying, "Keep calm, hold you're breathing, and dump them in the bin." Yes, a messy task, but he has been changing nappies with me for 3 years, and respectfully since 20 yr ago when his first son was born, those nappies never get closed/folded, never put in the bin, and the baby wipes are left next to the nappy station, and leaves it all. "Why don't you social distance yourself and throw away the nappy?"

"Are you keeping count? It's only 4,000 more to go!" AGHHHHHH!

Do not let the darkness of others hide the glow of your heart.

About the Author

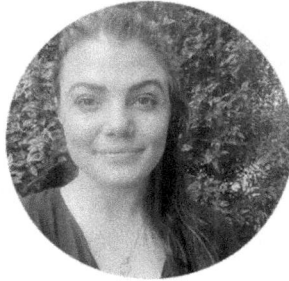

Aiesha Rowles-Oliver lives with her husband, Matt, and their two gorgeous kids and stepson in Mackay, Queensland, Australia.

She is continually on a journey of discovery in Herbal Medicine, passionate about her studies and health and wellness strategies, seeking solutions for her family's health and well-being, and gaining knowledge in many areas of energy healing for which to approach many topics.

She enjoys the Singin Bowl and other tribal instruments to elicit calm.

"Never do anything in a hurry; do everything in a calm spirit, even if chaos prevails."

Email: mdtcajc82@gmail.com

-ʌʌ→

Tanya Ruggeri

Fired Up!

What fires me up to do all that I do? I would rather live one day as a lion than one hundred years as a sheep. This is the most crucial quote you will read today. There was a time ten years ago when I wasn't fired up, yet had to act as if I was. Now, I am inspired by the person I have become. Another quote that has inspired me over the years is

'The difference between a winner and a loser is that the winner gets back up one more time.'

Pat Benetar sings *All Fired Up* as I fearlessly engage in my powerhouse morning routine. I lift weights in our home gym, The Cave, with my life partner Nekea and our little French bulldog Master ZaZu. He encourages us from the top of the

233

stairs, watching intently. We witness a thought bubble rising from his head, *"Do what scares you until it doesn't"*!

"We hear you ZaZu," we reply. He tilts his head and snorts with satisfaction! We all get back up, and we all keep going.

I was raised by a strong-to-the-core woman from Homebush, just a short drive from Mackay, Queensland, Australia. My Mums life started hard, she was born on her grandmother's bed in 1926 during the depression and war years, and they were tough times back then. Dad was a WWII return serviceman who immigrated to Australia from Italy when he was six years old and was a brilliant man.

An inventor, a future thinker, and a real Einstein to me.

I grew up with him reading me medical books and Encyclopaedias. I watched him invent numerous things over the years. My favorite was a pushbike with rear-view mirrors adorned with lights and horns! It was a dragster that looked very much fired up!

I went to an all-girls Catholic school and failed academically. I felt I wasn't designed for the school system. 'If you tell a fish to climb a tree, it will think it is dumb for the rest of its life.' I managed to attract plenty of the wrong type of attention. I was known as the class clown, but one lesson I quickly learned from the Nuns was the judicial Rattan Cane!

There were eight of us in our family.

My Five siblings were born and raised on the Sugar cane farm at Mt Charlton, and I was the number six child meaning there was a considerable age gap between me and my siblings I was born when Mum and Dad moved from the farm to town. I never lived on the farm but have been told many stories by my siblings. Farm life was hard, and they did it challenging, yet Mum and Dad always supported all children, even as adults. Our Italian heritage meant EATING - and lots of it. The food was all fresh, home-cooked meals. Dad was the master of spaghetti, and Mum was the 'old-fashion meat-vegetables-potatoes-type-of-cook.' The rule existed never to leave anything on the plate, no waste. Our parents were raised in times of *lack* and mentally stayed in it. Dad always said it must be an Italian thing if you weren't eating... "You were sick!" None of this Kentucky Fried Chicken I only ever got a whiff of as Dad sped by the KFC restaurant.

My childhood was littered with great moments; my love of skateboarding, bike riding, and my dogs. Those dogs, I would play dress-ups, but funny, horrors-of-horrors put ME in a dress now that was a different story altogether!! I would scream and cry as I only wanted to wear shorts and t-shirts and play with my guns and bow and arrows. Music turned out to be my form of communication, and I would break into a song to explain what I was trying to say. I was also known for acting and drumming and featured in a girl's band. Mum and Dad were strong humans, and great ethics were instilled within us, and as I reflect now, they remind me of "tough times never last, but tough people do" and that *eat-everything* food ethic.

My first shift towards a dark place began when I was hit with a whammy at nineteen, a critical event that changed me forever.

I suffered a fall, resulting in a fractured skull and a subdural hematoma, bleeding on the brain. I was left on a metaphorical cliff's edge with so many questions about why and how, but I was blessed to survive this and had to decide my future. That current path led me into an abyss, a way no one would choose to be on. Alcohol, smoking, nightclubs, and I just existed in a world I felt I did not belong or even understand.

A more recent descent is when my Mum, Dad, and brother all became terminally ill, and I still had to continue with my professional and personal life as if nothing was happening behind the scenes. It was like 'Charlie and Chocolate Factory' caring for the 3 them of us together. Those 10 years were long and arduous. However, I would not change a thing, and they have been my Angels since passing into the universe and have watched over me ever since.

My dad asked me the day before he passed, "Tanya, how can I ever thank you?" "Dad," I said, "you already have." I smiled. "You have loved me since I was born, cared for me all my life, and helped me become the caring person I am today. So it is you, Dad, that I should be thanking!"

Elevation arrived.

I visualized myself standing with both arms outstretched like an eagle, I fell forward in slow motion over the edge of the cliff. Falling, falling, but then the Universe caught me. I said to myself, "Let go and let the universe" Mum, Dad, and Tom's Angel wings caught me, now protect me, and have allowed me to settle. I am forever grateful they saw me, and now I'm never looking back. I feel elevated all day, every day.

Today, my results are on fire in building my Real Estate business, my passion for wellness and health, and my chosen sport, Powerlifting, and Bodybuilding. I keep reminding myself, "Tough times don't last, but tough people do." I find it humorous when told I am an overnight success and so lucky! Gosh!! I suppose the harder I worked, the luckier I got! I guess the magic lies within my fierce un-subtle daily steps every day for twenty-two years, day in and day out, my luminous affirmations, my continuing pathway in Real Estate, overcoming the six long years within my health struggles, and my transformation journey, and now my passion for inspiring others.

My more recent health journey got me, too: Bad habits can also seep in, and what you fear the most can happen, so be careful what you think and say to yourself, as your mind does not know the difference between true and false. A bunch of fears crept in from the dark days after my fall, which surprised me, as I was also very game and a big risk-taker, and all of a sudden, the fear of flying came out of nowhere! A compounding effect occurred. The result: I forgot about ME.

I became pre-diabetic, and my face and hair were full of Seborrheic Dermatitis, Rosacea, and other inflammatory diseases that arrived to plague me, along with circulation issues, joint pains, and weight gain. My petite frame didn't like carrying 110+ kilograms. I tried all the diets, and it was all BIG FAT LIES! In my opinion, the Food Pyramid is all upside down. I now eat according to my upside-down theory and not by my *eat-everything* parental ethics, and my life has changed for the better!

A business associate introduced me to Ketone supplement drinks. Nekea and I were considering gastric band surgery, and this ketone supplement was our last resort before venturing down that track. So thankfully, the ketones worked immediately, and we did not need surgery and have done this all 100% natural!

At least we could still eat and enjoy food on our ketones.

We lost a significant amount of weight, a whole person, to be exact! 80kg between us! Network Marketing has assisted us in many other ways, helping others win. We have made new friends who were inspirational to me, and I'm so proud of what I've become. The moment we tasted it, we knew it would change our life, it was as if the lights came on, and this, too, is what fired us up. I decided I wanted to be a bodybuilder. The newly sprouted inspiration filled my cup.

I can now easily lift my open house signs, get up at 3 am x 5 days a week for training, have my life and career all on track, and have a good family-work balance, and my mental energy and focus are spot on! Your mind is the most incredible power, so use it well. The point of having goals isn't really to achieve them but what you become on the way to them.

"Tanya Ruggeri," the headline read, "Owns her own Real Estate business in Mackay is known for taking her path".

I made the Courier Mail local newspaper! As one of Mackay's most 'Ripped Women'!

They had my headshot with my famous bicep post sitting under the headline, and my iconic 'muscle-flex-pose-in-red and orange-bikini-with-flaming-background' had me FIRED UP with great pride!

Most recently, I have been recognized as not only the 'Ripped but one of the most inspiring Business Women of Mackay.' You see, the problem is people are hated when they are honest and are loved when they are fake.

READ THAT AGAIN!

They said I would need steroids and could never do this naturally. They said I would need stomach surgery. They said I was too fat. They said I would end up with loose skin.

They said I would need a tummy tuck. They said a woman going through menopause couldn't do it. They said I was too old and wouldn't build muscle. They said I would need steroids; they also said I needed illegal fat strippers. They said I wasn't good enough for the stage and I should consider a transformation competition instead. They said it was not good for my joints or ligaments. They talked about me behind my back. They said I couldn't do it on Keto. They called me a snowflake, and they laughed at me. They rejected me. They abandoned me. They ghosted me, gaslighted me, and they bullied me. They were all wrong!

My achievements to date that inspire me:

1st U/63kg Qld States x Bench (APU)

1st Qld State Qualifiers 3 x lifts (APU)

1st Nth Qld Games 3 x lifts (APU)

1st Open Women Natural Physique (ANB)

1st Overall Natural Achievement Award (ANB)

HEAR ME WHEN I SAY THIS!

I WAS TOLD I'D NEVER GET THIS FAR, AND THEY WERE RIGHT, I GOT FURTHER!

Nothing will hit you harder than life itself. It doesn't matter how hard you get hit; it is about how much you can take and keep fighting and getting back up. It's how much you can suffer, keep moving forward, and still keep getting back up; that is the key. Interestingly, I never read a book through school until I was twenty-five. Now I'm obsessed as I even have my library at home and can have three books on the go at any one time, and now look at me, here I am now, writing my own!

I resonate with one particular book, The Purple Cow by Seth Godin; if you haven't read it, please do. While exploring many entrepreneurial skills in the book, he teaches you how to leverage the power of success in a field of brown cows. I have Purple-Cowed-Myself to my success! Your business needs to stand out like a purple cow in a herd of brown cows.

I visualize every day and always see the result in my mind because if you can see it, you will always hold it in your hands!

Overnight success? Back to that *LUCK* thing again.

TO ME, LUCK = Persistence, Hard Work, Sacrifice, Discipline, Passion, Risk, Disappointment, Failure, Fear & Doubt, and Criticism.

The problem with that quote is they don't see the years of sacrifice, the late nights, the early mornings, the going without, the fears, and the doubts. They only know the surface results; however, never think to dig deeper, look further, and walk a day in my shoes because if they did, they would put their boots straight back On! Others' views are fascinating, aren't they?

This is an exciting word, *YUK,* as I was told recently by one of our members in our private Facebook group that one of the recent pictures I posted was responded to as *YUK!* She said I was such a Poser!

So I said to her, "You think this pic is YUK? But do you want to know what even yuckier is?"

Getting up at three am every day to a desk full of admin and office work while everyone else is sleeping!

Now that's Yuk!

Watching others eat vast amounts of carbs, sweets, and junk food in front of me while I eat grilled skinless chicken and Broccoli! Working out and lifting hefty weights five days a week, I walk and do cardio daily! Five years ago, I could not tie my shoelaces because my stomach was too big and fat to bend over! Having a belly so big it touched the steering wheel. Five years ago, I had no energy and a body full of aches and pains before starting my fat loss journey. Now you want to know what's not that,

YUK? Feeling strong and healthy every day. Going from a size twenty-two to a size eight. Yes, I suppose I am a poser sometimes, as that's what trainee bodybuilders must learn to do and practice daily!

FIRED UP!

Allowing myself to relax, refresh and reconnect to myself, my environment and my gorgeous partner is vital too. What would you do right now, this very minute? Let me ask you this? If time and money weren't a problem.

Travel, change your career path, lose weight, take up a sport, buy your dream car, build a new home, or just help others with charity and giving to the homeless and poor? Just get fired up about it. Just KEEP GOING until you hold your results in your hands.

That is what a Lion does, not a sheep, be brave! Don't listen to others' nonsense!

My rocks in life are our fur babies ZaZu, Zeth, Moonshine the cat, and especially Nekea. We are always together in either Nekea's art studio, recovering in our sparkling pool, walking on the sandy beach, or in our library and gym or the home office working, as we run the businesses from *"Our Cave"* and of course, most afternoons in spent in our cardio room. We do everything from home.

Nekea and I locked eyes over fifteen years ago, and I knew instantly our path would be on the same trajectory moving forward. We work, work out, swim, meditate, not necessarily in that order, and do a blend of transformational practices and daily affirmations that are all unique and empowering. We love offering others access to glowing and nourished energy through these affirmations. I post most day's cartoon-style pictures of ZaZu and his thoughts bubbles next to my fired-up selfies so that others can think about areas of life they like to change, turn negative feelings into positive ones, and live their life with emotions and self-worth.

I had somehow convinced myself to improve my life after that dreadful fall at nineteen.

Monkey-Chatter between my ears still does exist to this day in there somewhere. As you're aware, I am also responsible for changing others' lives and helping them achieve their dreams, and I love it! I do this by selling clients' homes and assisting others with buying property.

With my reputation as a local independent business owner in my hometown, I also enjoy supporting other local businesses. I understand my clients very well, moving through my experience as a disgruntled buyer years ago. The property agents and their communication skills were horrific, and this changed my perspective and led me to whom I am today professionally. I treat people how I would like to be treated, with empathy and respect, with their best intention at the forefront of my mind. Gorgeous clients have stated that I have unparalleled knowledge of the Mackay property market, sold their houses concisely with 110% focus on them, and how inspiring I was in today's business world.

A dear client came to me after significant problems with another listing agent amid her terrible grief from losing her husband. I offered her great understanding, compassion, and care, unlike the service she had received previously, and it was evident to me that the funds tied up in this house were the legacy her husband had left her for her future. I had her financial lot in my hands, and I love that I was able to assist and set her up for life. I toss and turn more at night, thinking about my client's financial state than mine. Their financial crisis, I too understand so well, along with debt recovery with the ability to recognize when others simply need professional help along with selling their assets, is their only option. The stress and pressure I can relate to; this hits hard, and it's a problematic turn in life to take on alone - I've walked the minefield and been blown apart, and now others can follow me as I have traversed the Molotov cocktail of the Real Estate industry.

Realty deals with the Three- D's: Debt - Divorce - Death, and this is where the most empathy is needed, as I have been in these positions myself.

I find myself singing in the key of Fleetwood Mac, and when I hear a drum solo or drum groove, I play my invisible drumsticks in the air, reinstating my fire. Believe me, when I say you are capable of this too! You have the right and power to evolve. I am no longer the person I used to be before. The duality in what you before differed from the person you become and the *bloom* you transition through.

If I can do it, you can do it! You may not want to do everything I do, but I bet you have your dreams and goals inside of you that you have suppressed and are just screaming to get out!!

I love what I do! I DO ME FOR ME, with fire in my belly. I can help change lives, stand on stages and talk about my journey, write books, and inspire people along their journeys.

If I only assist one person to spread their wings and not fall, I've changed myself and the world. I'll leave you with my favorite verse. If you resonate and feel my fire, reach out to me. I'd love to connect with you.

The Starfish Story:
Original story by Loren Eisley

One day a man was walking along the beach when he noticed a boy hurriedly picking up and gently throwing things into the ocean.

Approaching the boy, he said, "Young man, what are you doing?"

The boy replied, "Throwing starfish back into the ocean. The surf is up, and the tide is going out. If I don't throw them away, they'll die".

The man laughed and said, "Don't you realize there are miles and miles of beach and hundreds of starfish? You won't make any difference!"

After listening politely, the boy bent down, picked up another starfish, smiled at the man, and said, "I made a difference to that one."

About the Author

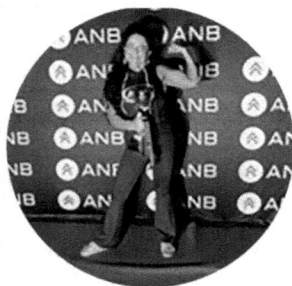

Tanya Ruggeri has been a Licensed Principle Real Estate Agent for 22 years and operates her own local independent business at Tanya Ruggeri Real Estate. Tanya is a Powerhouse in the Natural Powerlifting and Bodybuilding arena and a Ketones Health Endorser. She motivates and inspires many daily, hoping to inspire many-many more to achieve their dreams and goals.

When Tanya was offered the opportunity to participate and share her incredible story of inspiration with the world in the 'The New Rules Of Wellness' book series, she jumped at the chance to join the experts in this book. She knew that these experts who truly knew about health led from the heart and shared their stories of inspiration from a space of impact, and she wanted to be a part of it. She is a proper rising Phoenix who is fired up daily.

Website: www.tanyaruggerimeansbusiness.com.au
Instagram: @tanya_firedup_nattybodybulider
Facebook: www.facebook.com/groups/1686040618092841

-ⱳⱳⱳ→

Shirlz Russell

You are free to be different.

'I desire a life of unrealized hopes, unfulfilled wishes, and long-a-go-lost dreams,' SAID NO ONE EVER!

So how do we survive? How do we turn our dreams into reality? In my humble opinion, it's together. Supporting each other, building a tribe, a community. Ground zero can be a lonely place, a horrific space of self-doubt and loathing. When we rise from this emotional annihilation, thriving seems to dwarf the aforementioned 'nothingness.' If I can overcome self-limiting beliefs, non-deserving thought patterns, and total bankruptcy to re-address my life at a time when I felt all hope was lost – then I'm here to tell you, so can you! I know first-hand what it feels like to start again later in life when you're already supposed to have your SH*^T *together*. This humbling experience now sees me helping other women who are close to or thinking about retirement, who think it's too late to realize their dreams. I think the "difference" is defined by the energy we exhibit, we are what we repeatedly do, and we are what we resonate and connect with. Breaking free of 'the norm,' creating new rules and habits, taking consistent action, and setting new goals with an undying spirit to succeed. I am a female entrepreneur and have rebuilt a F'empire (no, I'm not swearing at you!) and supporting other women to build theirs too. Must I have constructed myself to be a change-maker as my social media account has recently been 'copied'---- silver lining? I'm *different* and *wonderfully excellent at NOT conforming!*

I worked hard, too willingly placed my trust and lost everything; that is my story. But man, did I learn a thing or two in the process!

You CAN go from having nothing to being utterly amazing, if you have the burning desire and believe. I'm that girl that once I make a decision, consider it done! This acute decisiveness has pained my partner Calvin, who sometimes takes FOREVER to make a decision (!). He often jokes that he has no idea how he bought a brand-new car and a business in the blink of an eye, not long after we first met. We are opposites in this and many other ways, and although he doesn't resonate or identify himself with the essence of who I am, he is extremely supportive and is bravely rolling with it... insert *LOVE HEART EMOJI*. He is at the center of my tribe, joined by my only child and inspiration - Olivia - and my Mum earthside, my Dad up above.

I'm pretty sure I scare the pants off my mother most days. She thinks I take on WAY too much, insert *EYE ROLL* (this eye-rolling is hereditary BTW; I'm always eye-rolling, Olivia is too, just ask my Mum), and don't get me wrong, I am indeed a busy girl, but there's a distinct difference with doing things that you love, versus doing things that you 'have' to. One is relatively stress-free. The other is not. I've worked insanely hard to create my incredibly fulfilling life. You see, my Mum and Dad experienced bankruptcy during my early teens, and when it all went pear-shaped for me, the thing I struggled with the most initially was how I could have let myself follow in their footsteps; I'd lived through their struggle first-hand and have since witnessed them work hard and yet never fully recover financially.

From those early days, I was surrounded by a real FEAR connection around money - my parents never again invested in property, as they didn't want to risk losing it all over again. They had built a sizable portfolio before losing it all, along with the business they had built from scratch. I'm confident their early successes is where my passion for both property & business began. Where they had developed a fear around investing, my fall from grace instead ignited a passion for rebuilding, never giving up on my dreams or letting fear hold me back - that will never be me. Historically, every decision made around money and finances from that point forward was seen as a massive risk. Recognizing this debilitating connection has allowed me to change my narrative.

I often have that feeling that everything is my fault, Or that I've failed. Generally because I've chosen to take on ALL the responsibilities! A perfect example is making sure everyone is fed - I love to cook (and love to eat too!), but I've recently come to realise that it's actually not MY responsibility to feed and water my partner - he is an adult and can actually feed himself - and don't get me wrong, I'm the one stuck in this pattern - he is completely ok with it - but the old traditional sentiment from my upbringing keeps me cocooned in a web of old habits and testaments; that's what my mum did - that's what women do, right? Man-pleasing? My father was a powerful man, and I constantly sought his approval as an only child. My new wellness rule is to PERMIT MYSELF, to allow myself to be myself, to be proud of myself, to be my own biggest fan - I don't need approval from an external source.

As women, we are genetically ingrained with that notion. It's also true that women usually assume the carer's role in any given situation, whether an unpaid role or the lowest-paying position (outside of volunteering!), whether at home, in the office, or a team environment. All this sentiment ultimately culminated in doing what I do now. I am the founder of Build Your F'empire. I am a property investment coach, helping women (and a few good men !) to build wealth through property. I have also developed an online platform to educate, support, mentor, and assist women to empower themselves and build a stable, independent financial future.

By default, I have become a mentor, especially to women in business or those looking to build a business. I am passionate about championing other women's successes and empathizing when they make mistakes - as this is our most beautiful opportunity to grow - and spreading the ideology of an abundance mindset to all who will listen. In life, we can choose between viewing the world as abundant or limited in terms of love, relationships, wealth and resources.

In life, our mindset determines which road we travel on. One road is paved in scarcity, and the other is filled with abundance at every turn. At any moment, we can choose to change which route we want to travel on.

The scarcity pathway leads us to experience a life not fully lived, a life that can only be described as a pedestrian - a little like my opening statement! Overflowing with adverse solid reactions like the high tide that creates waves in a rock pool, not to mention the countless missed opportunities and experiences.

Those that choose to walk along the path of abundance experience a completely different life. Opting to live life fully, exuding happiness, generous by nature, creative and inspirational. Taking full advantage and enjoying the wave of opportunities that come their way, along with memorable experiences.

Having nothing was a humbling experience, seemingly devoid of all hope. Like so many women, being given the short end of the stick has financially left me in such a vulnerable position. Lots of women I work with come through a divorce and feel like they've been blindsided. Only then, when it's too late, they realize just how dependent they have become on their spouse, that their income alone is insufficient to buy their own home. How many men are encouraged to stay home or consider returning to work part-time once they start a family, essentially taking on that unpaid 'carer's role' in the family? The knock on effect on a woman's financial position when starting a family is a huge handicap that is often overlooked in these situations. They are often victims of the gender pay gap, they may suffer financial and business losses, lack superannuation due to starting a family as mentioned above, and find themselves struggling to pay the bills, unable to see the light at all. Arguably, our male counterparts are usually positioned better and have a much higher overall financial outlook heading into retirement, even if they have been through the exact same asset relocation program (divorce!). My courses cover various topics, from an emotional twist on money matters, goal setting, the magic behind a great and functional budget, how to become financially independent, and heaps of fun money management tricks.

IT IS WHAT IT IS - GO WITH IT, ROLL WITH IT. ALL WILL BE OK.

One day I changed; I lost my dad in 2019. He and I were pretty similar in personality, very close, but we would often butt heads; I, on the cusp of both Aries and Taurus versus him, a Scorpio. I guess you could say we were both a little headstrong! Ours was a relationship of fire, never holding back, but with so much underlying love. He was my go-to person, sometimes I'd call him 10 times a day. He was my sounding board, my voice of reason, and the holder of that 'approval' I always sought. I still can't delete his number from my phone. It killed me inside to see him give up on his dreams, a strong person who mentally gave up and his body eventually followed. This was a catalyst to take control of my life and create the right balance for ME. He was unwell for so long. I don't want that; I want to live in the now.

Being completely in control of my time, saying 'yes' to attending school or sporting events for my daughter and having both the flexibility and finances to afford taking a trip each and every school holidays is my lifeblood; spending quality time together exploring this wonderful world on each new and exciting adventure. This is my new normal. This is me now taking control of and 'approving' for myself.

The wellness rules I grew up with were to assist others no matter what, always love and support others, and help them to help themselves before themselves.

Even when they had nothing, I have memories of my parents always helping other people; it's an innate quality to serve in some way, and I also teach Olivia. Being awarded the Spirit of Jesus, award was one of my proudest mummy moments. She's a beautiful little helper at home and is constantly being asked to lead the way and help out by her teachers at school. Resoundingly, her report cards talk of her being kind, looking after her mates and being a genuinely good human. So proud. I've realized, though, that we can live the life we want to lead and do what makes us happy while still supporting others. We can do this AND put ourselves first. There's a distinct difference.

My pet peeve is non-responders, people who don't call me back. This is another area where my partner and I are very different. He has SO MANY unread messages. It makes me anxious just looking at them. My inbox must be cleared; anything left there has yet to be actioned. That way, I know I've done everything. I'm also very organised and need everything in its place. Being able to pop out for a few hours through the day or schedule a full day away from the office is what makes being your own boss so rewarding. Yes, I might work until late some nights and do a few hours here and then when on holidays, but I always manage to get things done AND do the things I want to do too. I no longer subscribe to what others deem 'normal.' Those with a 9-

5 job will often say how unhealthy it is to be working late at night, early mornings or whilst on holidays. Tell me, friend, do you take annual holidays for up to 12 weeks? Do you do lunch and coffee dates and attend all of the networking and personal development programs you'd like to? Yeah, I didn't think so!

I can live a minimal existence, and there is nothing specific I HAVE to have or can't live without. However, I like the finer things in life and am a 5-star gal all the way. I also love getting back to basics and roughing it every now and then. I'm the go-camping-with-nothing girl; I don't take much other than the bare necessities, everyone has all their sh*t, and I just have my tent and bedding, that's it. So many camping adventures that have offered so much joy—tops up my cup; Homestead at Lotus Creek locally on holidays, then off to Airlie Beach up here in the Whituandays, and living it up. We Dine at Sorrentos—the most amazing Italian food and seafood in a stunning location overlooking the water.

Next—was China. Such a highlight for us all. I was asked recently what I would do more if I had all the time and money. Travel. To explore the world as I feel I haven't explored enough of yet. Different cultural experiences made me realize we are little dot's, all of us but just a spec. "You are not a drop in the ocean; you are an ocean in a drop. That's deep!"-Rumi. Let's just be ourselves–for who gives a f*ck, we are tiny things, why conform? What is conformity? It all make me not care about what others think, so much hardship in the world, we are so lucky and can make decision, we get to decide what to eat. I did decide what I wanted to eat in China—but there were a few surprises.

Sitting in a lovely restaurant, people bustling around us, the environment was bustling. We had not mastered understanding the Chinese language—every moment was an adventure. We ordered by pointing at words on the menu, as our fingertips parused the items, stopping at random meals. There was an aura of excitement; what were we going to get? My bowl arrived; it was a kind of soup. Items floating and swirling and smelled divine. I placed my spoon, stirred, and nearly fainted when I saw CHICKEN BEAKS float to the surface. Eating the lightweight keratin I know is a hair, skin and nails remedy, but seriously? Looking at the little nostrils, Ironically, I couldn't breathe myself, a real WOW moment! Another WOW moment was the Great Wall of China. This opened my eyes to the magnitude of what's possible. An idea and to believe it and get it done. Not to mention my walking up to the top of the wall, the 5 hour trek I had to embrace the Tao energy to get that job done! Shanghai and the Terracotta Warriors—another version of myself was born that trip—anything is possible.

Next? Japan. Olivia has embraced entrepreneurial energy and created a dehydrating fruit business to facilitate achieving her Japan dream realized. Another proud Mummy moment!

Today, I asist others to bloom where they are planted.

Conversationalists all look particularly regal tonight; trusty friends in black tie, speeches prepared, and the band ready to perform. The guest list for the 'Shades Of Women' event in Mackay, full of kickass women, consists of generous business owners, sponsors, volunteers, and the support is indispensable. Acknowledging the trauma and triumphs of some truly inspirational women, victims and survivors of DV—such a gorgeous night. My table place setting 'Table 8 - Build Your F'empire" and Fearless & Wild earrings bonbonniere, I've created a community and gathered businesses around the premise of females supporting each other and thriving, and we all now sit at the same table chinking champagne glasses. I am the founder of Build Your F'Empire, a Female-supporting-female business and support group of entrepreneurs, a women-focused initiative.

Local community, community group supporting building their empire. Support local community, board member of the Australian Street Aid Project (ASAP) Charity. Bridging the services gap for homelessness in Mackay. This is close to my heart and quite representative of what I do. I find it incredibly alarming that the fastest-growing demographic for homelessness in Australia is women aged 55+, divorced, and unable to support themselves financially.

Reach out to this silver-lining gal; there is a reason; let's make it a good one. I love to start a conversation with you, see how I can support you best. Our feminine power is within our ability to stand out, not conform. #neversettleforless Talented women rise; let's be there for each other. With me, Pink hair, 52 pairs of shoes, and Dopamine dressing (Dressing in colour for those who don't know)—Being a Queen with the strength of a warrior.

'Your biggest weakness is when you give up; your most significant power is when you try one more time' - Marie Angel.

About the Author

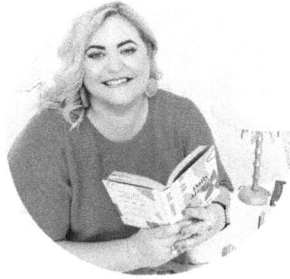

Shirlz Russell is the founder of Build Your F'empire, a community based support network and resource hub for women looking to take control of their finances. She is a well-respected coach and mentor to women in business, and her clients include women from all walks of life. In her primary role as a property investment coach, she specializes in providing a 'done for you' approach for women who are switched on and ambitious and are looking for ways to get ahead, and beyond.

She and her partner Calvin reside in sunny North Queensland, where together they run other Entrepreneurial ventures, 'Kombi Keg Whitsundays' in their spare time. Shirlz' daughter Olivia and Mum Monica live with them and their fur babies in their resort style home where they love to entertain and enjoy the tropical lifestyle.

Website: buildyourfempire.com.au
Email: shirlz@buildyourfempire.com.au
Facebook: www.facebook.com/groups/buildyourfempiregroup

-vvvv→

Lauren Thompson

From a young age, I knew I didn't fit in. The funny way that people looked at my parents, who were much older than the other kid's parents, and the way that teachers would lament the fact that I spent more time gazing out of the window than I did doing actual schoolwork, made it clear that I was seen as an oddball.

In class, I found my mind wandering into the worlds I'd found myself escaping into instead sitting to attention and listening to the facts and figures taught in class. I found inspiration in the worlds created by J.K. Rowling, Tolkien, and George Lucas; I was a huge nerd.

My parents weren't worried that I didn't fit the mold of an ideal student. My father told teachers I was just a "deep thinker." It wasn't until secondary college that I discovered my love for English and writing. I had book reviews I wrote featured in the school newsletter. My teachers started to say I had a "gift for words." When I was 15 years old, I decided to become a writer and share my stories with the world, no matter how impossible it seemed.

For so long I had been going through the motions since graduating from university. I'd been working as a freelance writer and plodding here and there at my book. The sun beat down on my brow through the glass door as I sat at my desk, typing furiously, getting scenes down quickly while the hows and whys of the plot kept escaping me. I killed off a character in my earliest drafts, inserted a villain that my beta reader wasn't taking seriously, and wondered if they were even in the story. I wanted to write a story about a girl who embarked on a journey to a land few had ever traveled to, discovering truths about her world and herself. But all the working parts of the story just weren't flowing together.

Again, I felt like the girl who couldn't get things together. The one who was always behind and wasn't as together or as "accomplished" as she should be. The one desperately trying to prove she was "enough" through long work hours. I hadn't changed, and I wasn't "enough." At least, that's what I told myself as a furiously typed-out words for a narrative that never seemed to come together. I'd shown pieces of the story to my beta reader, and the villain wasn't quite working for them. There was still a missing ingredient. Something I couldn't quite put my finger on as to what exactly was missing.

Only when I applied for a volunteer role where I needed to obtain a copy of my birth certificate did a piece of my own story become more apparent. One day my father sat me down, and we had a conversation that redefined my life. He told me he needed to have a conversation with me that was long overdue. I had never seen my birth certificate before and was about to for the first time. He sat down in his recliner, the light shining off his balding head. He looked smaller and frailer than ever before, and I made a couple of jokes to lighten the mood, knowing deep down that he was about to reveal information that would rock my entire world, and I wasn't ready for it. He finally cleared his throat and told me the story of his younger brother, my Uncle Donald, a complicated man with many demons who never seemed content.

He fell in love with a married woman who was devout Catholic and married to an influential man in their community. But the pair wished to be together. They were just waiting for the right time to make it official. They were not ready to make their relationship official, and her husband was influential in the community. The brothers had grown up in an environment where they could only depend on one another for support, with their mother sending them away for their safety after their father lost his temper with the children one too many times, and the oldest child, my father had stepped into the role of parent from a young. As a result, his younger brother had always looked to him to fix any problem he encountered. So, when he asked his older brother to drive from Victoria to Queensland because of an emergency, my father didn't hesitate. The moment my father and mother arrived in a direct children's park in the dead of winter as the sun went down. My mother and father huddled together for warmth as the winds whipped around them, and a solemn silence fell over the pair as my uncle told them the story of his affair of how his lover was now pregnant with a girl—me.

The person I'd believed to be my uncle was my biological father; the man I'd called my father all my life was my uncle.

I went numb as the man I now realize was my adoptive father spoke. His words flooded my mind, and moments from my life where I never felt I belonged replayed like an old recording. That nagging feeling that constantly tore at the back of my mind while growing up suddenly made so much more sense. My adoptive father had once said when I was growing up that having me was the "best decision he and your mother ever made." It should have been evident for several reasons.

Growing up, they gave me a protective (and sometimes overprotective) environment, taking me on trips worldwide to provide me with the best start in life and showering me with attention.

"I'm a coward," my adoptive father muttered, tearing me from my thoughts and tearing through my heart. When my eyes finally met his, I saw the look of a man consumed by guilt. He regretted not telling me sooner, and he and my adoptive mother had apparently talked about how to say to me many times, but they'd never quite known how. And thinking back on the story and looking at all the pieces of the puzzle that have now fallen into place, I can't help but understand why.

Only a week after my birth, my biological mother left on a plane back to Queensland with my biological father, never returning or contacting me again. My biological mother was wary of making contact with me, lest she is excommunicated from her church and community, not only for having an affair but for having a child out of wedlock. Any desire to see me or have me in her life was ultimately overridden by fear of what her family and community would think of her actions.

Although, after pouring through old legal documents, my biological father wanted to take custody of me, in he was never able to gain custody of me, and wanted to block my adoptive father from adopting me at the time, simply because he held too much spite towards his older brother to let him "win" even if that is what was deemed best by the courts. I'm told he saw me once briefly as a toddler but decided never to see me again after that, and he was consumed by his alcoholism and his past demons and died while still a relatively young man. My biological parents knew where to find me and stayed in my adoptive parent's home while waiting for my birth. However, they ultimately rejected being a part of my life because of their fears about how I would impede on their public reputation and personal demons. That's not easy to tell a young child or even a teenager. And my biological father was well-known as an unstable and aggressive man who never stayed anywhere or with anyone long. In my adoptive parent's minds, knowing him, or even knowing of him, would have thrown the security they were trying so hard to provide for me into chaos. But now my father sat before me as an adult woman and vowed to answer any question I might have, knowing this moment was long overdue.

As much as I have moments where I wish they could have told me sooner, I ask myself how I would suggest to a young child in my care that their parent was related to me, but they couldn't and wouldn't be a part of your life. I would struggle to explain such a thing to a vulnerable child. And if I had known, I would have felt like a source of shame to my birth parents, one they'd had to hide away in another part of the country so they could continue with the rest of their lives. After I had run through the labyrinth of emotions that comes with finding out you're adopted, I went to a new appreciation of the family I was accepted into rather than the one I was born into.

The time I was working on obtaining my Master's degree was marked by restless nights and the fear of losing my mother. My mother suffered from COPD (Chronic Obstructive Pulmonary Disease), and her struggles to breathe nearly took her life when I started my Master's degree. Her movements became slower and slower over time. Just as I was beginning my Master's degree and my career in freelance writing, she was slowly slipping from my life. She fell into an induced coma for two weeks. I was simply going through the motions for those two weeks. Waking, eating, working, and going to bed. I felt like I was on autopilot.

After two weeks had passed, the doctors took me and my family aside. She was still in a coma. They asked us if we wanted to take her off life support. We all exchanged looks of silent agreement, unable to say the words we were thinking aloud. Mum was going to die. We told the doctors to take her off the life support. However, my mother took slow, steady breaths and looked around in raw confusion. I said so much and so little to her the moment she came. I can't remember what I said or what she said, just the sheer relief from talking with her. It took many months for her to recover to the point where she could return home. She lived for three more years. It was only 6 months after she'd attended my graduation ceremony after receiving my Master's degree that her movements began to slow in a way that was all too familiar, and she became bedridden.

While lying in bed and inhaling her puffer, my mother asked me how I was going with my novel, which would become Isle of Dragons. I told her I was progressing and she would see it one day. Even as the light seemed to fade from her eyes, she offered me a weak smile and declared that it would be "something great." However, just hours after that conversation, she fell into a coma, where her breath became ragged, and she fell into another coma.

My breath began to catch, and my hands trembled slightly. My family and I knew she would not come out of the coma this time.

"Do you want to come?" My father had asked me softly over the phone just as the ambulance arrived to take her to the hospital for what we all knew would be the last time.

How quickly the word "no" tumbled from my mouth shocked me. Fear ran through my body that froze me in place when he asked that question. He told me he understood and told me he'd stay in touch and call anytime I wanted. But I still carried a deep shame gripping my chest, but the thought of sitting in the hospital beside her, waiting for life to sleep away, shook me in a way few things had up to that point in my life. The ambulance had taken my mother in the early morning hours, and I spent the rest of the day walking in a dream-like state, unable to work or do anything other than sit and wait for the inevitable.

I stared at the clock bleary-eyed as I sat at my kitchen table with a mug of peppermint tea. It was 12:45 pm. My mother lay in the hospital, still in a coma. I picked up my phone and called a friend I knew had lost her mother at a young age, and the only advice she had for me was to let my mother know how I felt before it was too late. After our conversation, I took a deep breath and finally summoned the courage to do what I knew I should have done all along. I rang my father and asked him if he could hold the phone up to my mother, the only mother I'd ever known; goodbye and I love you. And at that moment, while still trapped in a coma, a tear rolled down her cheek before she took one last breath and faded from the world. My father sat in silence a moment before describing to me what had just happened. I closed my eyes and sat back in my chair, letting the reality that she was gone wash over me. Even in a coma, my mother had waited for me to say goodbye one last time before taking her.

After that, I began to write and write, determined to fulfill my promise to get my books out into the world. I finally saw my first novel, the Isle of Dragons, in print a few years later. I'd done it. And little by little, I've created more stories that give inspiration and hope to those who may feel like they don't fit in or are "behind" in life.

My stories revolve around characters discovering who they are and who don't quite fit into conventional expectations and tick certain boxes of how people are "supposed to be" while discovering community and connections in the unlikeliest places. The Isle of Dragons series hits on many themes of striving to find acceptance and breaking against expectations of who they should be. Jade is a creative spirit who loves magic and creating things, but she's trapped in an environment where magic is frowned upon and considered a significant crime. When her father is taken from her, she embarks on a journey to find him, meeting many people she thinks of as family and embracing parts of herself she was too afraid to before. Jade rebuilds her life and identity, expands her family, and creates a new home for herself, gradually discarding the parts she felt she had to hold onto to feel accepted by society. Jade expresses my journey to no longer feeling "stuck" in life due to not fitting into conventional ideas of who they should be.

Jade and her rival Kaylen embark on a journey of self-discovery where they learn to accept the parts of themselves that they are taught are wrong and begin to find acceptance with people outside of the restrictive environments they were born into. Kaylen is an orphan and Jade's childhood friend who turns against Jade when faced with the choice of helping her friend or jeopardizing her position in the royal army. I have far more in common with Kaylen and her journey of self-acceptance than I am comfortable admitting! But both Jade and Kaylen mirror parts of my journey and relationship with my sense of self. They are both different sides of the same coin. Jade expands on her idea of home and family and learns to let go of the notion that things should be specific, while Kaylen gives into the pressures around her and betrays her principles so she can feel a sense of belonging. But she's forced to reassess her views and ideas about who her true family is and where her loyalties lie.

My novella, *The Prince and the Witch,* revolves around a young prince who feels unprepared for the expectations to be a strong and uncompressing ruler like his father. His journey takes him on the path of discovering new ways of looking at the world that he never considered before. By the end of the book, he is ready to take on the mantle of leadership, but in a different manner than what was expected of both his father and society. He eventually embraces the people and things that he was taught to fear and embraces the parts of himself he was taught to resent. Edward's journey mirrors my journey to understand myself and embrace my identity.

It took some time to understand it and put it into practice, but I found my passion and purpose in reaching out to those who might need it through words. I write for the kids who struggle to fit in with other kids and feel like something is wrong because they don't fit into the idea of what they should be like in one way or another.

About the Author

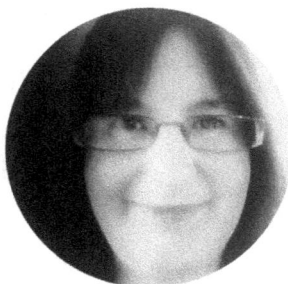

Lauren Thompson is a freelance writer of fantasy young adult books. She lives on the south coast of Victoria with her partner and dog, a beagle named Sasha. She has a Bachelor of Arts Degree in Professional and Creative Writing and a Master of Arts Degree in Writing and Literature. Previously working with the Society of Women Writers Victoria (SWWV).

She writes under the pen name L. A. Thompson and has released 3 fantasy novels, two of which are part of the *Isle of Dragons* series, first published in 2019—runner-up in the 2020 Readers Favorite Book Award. Future installments will be released in late 2023. She has written a standalone novella called *The Prince and the Witch*.

Website: https://la-thompson.com

Where to buy my books:

www.amazon.com/Isle-Dragons-1-L-Thompson-ebook/dp/B0B85XJS29
www.amazon.com/Prince-Witch-L-Thompson-ebook/dp/B09YYKSYRW

-ᗯᐯᐯ→

Amanda Tremlett

CFS: From Discovery to Recovery

Discovery

I sat at my kitchen table, crying, I realized my life was over.
After two hours of staring at the floor, taking in the news that
this fit and active, always on the move, single Mum had CFS. I
did not know how to compute this new information. My
dreams were shattered, and my future was gone.

It began in October 1997. I had flu, or so I thought, and I was
not improving. For the next three years, I had multiple doctor's
appointments to get to the cause of my aches and pains and
continuous fatigue. The doctor decided that I was depressed. I
knew I was not, but he would not hear me. I was frustrated
and upset and was looking for a solution that was not coming.
I decided to try a different doctor.

After a year of getting to know him, I gained enough courage to discuss my symptoms. I was nervous that I would not be heard again and would be labeled depressed. I opened up and told him what my previous doctor had said. I shared my symptoms, and he listened carefully. When I had finished, I waited anxiously for his response. I was thinking *here it comes*. You're depressed.

It's all in your head. You're lazy. There's nothing wrong with you.

Which one are you going to say?

What he said surprised me. I was not depressed. He said the symptoms sounded like ME (CFS), but it could be another condition that presented with similar symptoms. He referred me to a consultant to figure out what was going on. It had taken four years to get to this point. I felt a sense of relief. I could relax a little because I knew I was on the right road to discovering the truth. Once I knew what was wrong with me, I could figure out what to do with it.

After blood tests ruled out other conditions, I was diagnosed with CFS. It felt good to know the cause finally. I had a starting point to understand and manage what was happening to me. Although my moment of joy vanished as quickly as it had appeared when he explained that I was unlikely to recover as I had been sick for more than four years. I was heartbroken. Bring on the kitchen table, crying, and floor staring!

At subsequent visits, I was offered antidepressants to suppress the symptoms or painkillers for the pain. I declined both. The consultant had previously explained that I would need to monitor what it was doing to manage the condition. Taking either medication would make this impossible as the symptoms would be masked. I had no issue taking medication if it was proven to aid recovery, but I was not willing to accept them if it would not cure me. As time passed, I realized I had to change how I viewed my health. Focusing on how miserable life had become was not the answer now I had chronic pain, muscle fatigue, and a brain that no longer functioned much of the time. I needed to do something to make this experience bearable, even though it seemed impossible. I began researching CFS to learn what was happening to my once-healthy body.

I learned that it might be a misdiagnosed thyroid problem, a zinc deficiency, or a magnesium deficiency. I might even be suffering from Lyme Disease or Epstein-Barr virus. The list went on! There were 'man in the street' experts who concluded that I was 'lazy,' 'depressed,' or just plain 'making it up.' As a formerly fit and active person, that hurt the most. Why would someone so determined to do well in life create a condition that left them lethargic and incapable of the simplest tasks such as eating and speaking? Dealing with the symptoms was terrible enough. To be judged as a fraud hurt more. There were just as many therapies, solutions, and drugs that suggested they could cure me too. I studied all their claims, but they did not fit with what I knew about what was happening to my body.

It was hard to stay positive; my social life had pretty much ended, friends had moved on, and I struggled to work out how to manage myself, my family, and my home between relapses. There simply were not enough hours in the day when I was well enough to function. I felt defeated. I cried a lot. I was frustrated, angry, and hurt that the universe had dealt me this terrible hand. An intentional analogy, I never could grasp card games!

So, with my brain kaput and my body broken, I embarked on a journey of discovery. How would I live with chronic pain and limited energy and soothe the spirit that desperately wanted life to be the way it used to be or, at least, something similar to it? I bought myself a wheelchair, put it in the corner of the room, and told myself, 'You are not going to end up in that!' I was going to find the cause, I was going to find the solution, and I was going to get well. I concluded that if I believed it enough, it would happen. For the first time, I had hope.

The in-between days

And so my transformation began. I researched CFS. I studied my symptoms to learn about other possible diagnoses. I talked to my consultant. I spoke to a psychologist. I researched every detail to discover how to have the best life possible without giving in to negativity. My journey through my new reality began with simplifying everyday tasks to reduce stress and conserve energy for things that mattered. I learned that my positive attitude would determine the key to my success.

Sometimes mealtimes were challenging. I did not have the physical energy to lift my hand to my mouth, and I could not work out how to make a sandwich. When my cognitive function was low, I would not force it. If I could not work out how to make a sandwich, I would eat the ingredients as they were, two slices of bread followed by a chunk of cheese. Did it matter that it was not packaged in a pretty sandwich package? No, it did not. When it reached my stomach, it would still break down and provide me with the same nutrients. A whole new way of looking at the world had started. My new way of thinking powered everything I did.

Over time I found solutions to most problems, like getting up and down stairs (I am glad nobody was around to video that!).

I slept on the stairs once when I was too exhausted to make the whole journey! I also learned to make toast using the grill without burning it every time! I stopped worrying about things that did not matter and focused on what I did have and could do rather than on things that were missing. On days when I was confined to bed, I would watch cloud formations and think about how varied and impressive they were. I spent a lot of time looking at the sky! I saw things other people missed, like rainbows, a circum-horizontal arc, and a circumzenithal arc. I could tell when the weather was going to change. On days when I could get out of bed, I would be grateful for being able to stand and take small steps. I treasured the feeling of the wool carpet under my feet. It felt soft and comforting. I had learned to be grateful for the little things; there was beauty in all of it. Life was looking more positive as I changed my perception of it.

With my newfound positive thinking and the simplification of tasks, I had a bit more time to do the things I wanted. I started a new journey into higher education. I studied part-time to manage the workload and felt positive doing something productive. I had an exam in my first semester. I was allowed to use a PC to type my answers as handwriting increased the pain in my hands. During the exam, I discovered that I was struggling to type letters in the correct order. I was assessed by a psychologist, who said I had indicators of Dyslexia. Still, they could not conclude it was dyslexia because the CFS symptoms contributed to my problems. The psychology report led to four more assessments. I was diagnosed with Dyspraxia and visual stress, and there was a 90% chance that I had ADHD. In light of these results, it was later decided that I probably did have dyslexia.

This was a lot to take in!

It explained a lot but was scary too. I now understood why I did not like reading for long periods, walked into things, got bored quickly, and needed to be active. Armed with this knowledge, I began to study how these conditions impacted my cognitive function, physical health, and mental and emotional well-being. I learned that I could not multitask, could not process lots of information quickly, would likely have problems falling asleep, and felt exhausted was highly probable. I did not have a light bulb moment yet, but I was getting there. One piece of the puzzle was still missing. It would take a few more years before the switch was flipped, and the light would come on like a million LEDs!

In 2010, I had a breakdown; the suppressed memory of a traumatic experience from my teenage years returned to haunt me. Lying dormant for almost 30 years, it raised its ugly head and terrified me! Here began a new challenge, PTSD and its multifaceted drama! Flashbacks, intense physical pain, nightmares, and an inability to think or sometimes sleep. The universe has given me much to research and understand over the years. PTSD was no different, and as I did, EUREKA! The light came on, the sun came out, the last piece of the jigsaw slotted into place, and I saw the cause, the solution, and a way out of chronic disability!

PTSD causes fatigue, headaches, brain fog, and physical pain. I looked into solutions to overcome it and the trauma I had experienced. I tried out different things and developed a solution that worked. As I unraveled the past and implemented the solutions I had learned to live with neurodiversity, I saw my life and health change. I began my journey back to total health with my new collated wisdom.

I shared my learning with others who struggled with CFS but was saddened by the response I received. Some were intrigued and wanted to know more but were unwilling to work to recover; others did not want to get well because they enjoyed the attention they received from those around them while sick. My excitement waned until I realized I cannot be the only person with CFS who wanted to get well. I told myself that one day I would tell my story, and here I am today, sharing what was a 21-year journey for me in the hope that I can help others recover their health sooner.

Recovery

Recovery is only possible once we know what we are recovering from. Chronic Fatigue Syndrome describes one symptom but does not describe what it is. CFS results from a set of complex factors coming together to create chaos.

The first thing to recognize is that CFS is a lie that keeps faking. It is not a physical illness. It presents with physical symptoms, but your body is not the problem. Certain people are more susceptible to developing CFS. When researching, I discovered that those with CFS were autistic, had ADHD, dyslexia, dyspraxia or visual stress, or multiple close family members had these challenges. How the brain functions with these conditions makes it more likely that a person will develop CFS. I discovered that CFS results from unresolved psychological issues and neurodevelopmental challenges that are not managed effectively.

Stating that CFS is partly psychological has been challenging for some CFS sufferers to accept when I have shared it with them. Symptoms like brain fog are caused by unprocessed information backing up in the brain; often, this is trauma or unresolved issues from an earlier time in their life. Also, the pain felt throughout the body results from trauma from the past that has not been processed and the brain being overloaded and needing a break. The brain is the control center for our nervous system; when it is overloaded, it sends out faulty messages to the body.

It is screaming,' Help! I'm stressed! I can't deal with any more stimuli! Please let me go somewhere dark and quiet for a break! I need to recover!'

When someone says,' It's all in your head! ' they are correct, but not how they believe. If you have CFS and have been beating yourself up, thinking you are lazy and not sick, STOP! Take a breath, and tell yourself, 'I am not functioning well at the moment because my brain is crammed full of stuff; it is under stress and needs to declutter.' Give yourself a moment to feel that validation. After years of not being understood or supported, I support you.

You will get the idea if you think of your brain as a computer processing lots of information quickly. A new, up-to-date PC can quickly process incoming information and has the memory capacity to handle it. Those with ADHD, autism, or other neurodevelopmental wiring do not have the same setup. We have the equivalent of a ten-year-old PC. Have you ever tried to use an older piece of technology in the present? It crashes, it slows up and stops, we get mad, we get frustrated, we yell, 'Why won't you work! Please work! I need to get this done!' If you have CFS, do you recognize this? Have you said this to yourself when the CFS has ramped up, you know you have things to do but nothing left to work with? Your brain is the equivalent of that old piece of technology. Give it a break, be easy on yourself, and relax. You are not the problem. Your brain is not the problem; how you are using your brain is the problem. When you figure out how it is wired, you can function in the present and learn how to become CFS-free.

CFS often starts with flu-like symptoms. I was constantly sick when I had CFS. I was run down and picked up viruses regularly. I believed that I had an immune system problem. This is true to some extent. When overloaded, the brain cannot run the immune system effectively. The immune system does recover once pressure on the brain to function beyond capacity ends. As I recovered from CFS, I was sick less often and recovered more quickly. My immune system usually functions now.

I have been CFS-free since 2018. When the light came on, and I recognized what CFS was, I could reverse the process. I learned how to rest my brain, deal with the overload, and function in the present with the wacky brain I have. I now use my brain efficiently and effectively to have the life I want. I run my own business helping clients to simplify their lives, reduce stress, and prevent burnout while creating time, space, and energy to do the things they love. If you are unhappy, if you want relief, if you are tired of being sick and tired, then embrace the fact that you can have the life you want too; all you need is the knowledge and the desire to do it.

The knowledge is that your brain is not like other brains. You will see a change once you start using it how it should be used. Learning to love your neurodiversity can take time, but there are positives to being different. Richard Branson has dyslexia. He is innovative and creative; his achievements are multifaceted. Many entrepreneurs have ADHD. We see the world differently and have talents others do not have. We have unique talents that we use to contribute great things to society. Being different is not a curse it is a blessing. It is only a problem if we believe it is. We process information differently, and once we learn what we can, we can change ourselves and our lives and influence the world around us. The desire to heal is within you.

If I can do it, so can you.

If you have survived CFS to this point, living daily with chronic pain and fatigue, you can recover. Embrace the reality that you are special and unique; the world needs you and your talents. The world needs your story of recovery. Go into the world from this point onwards with the power of knowing you can heal. The journey towards a new and brighter, more energy-filled future is there for the taking.

I have given you a lot to think about it. You will need time to absorb it. When you are ready, reach out and connect; let us travel this road together!

About the Author

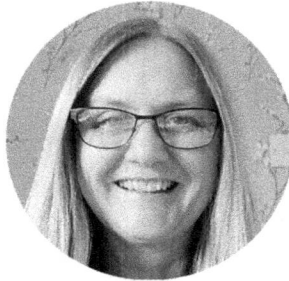

Amanda Tremlett is a Simplicity Strategist, Neurodiversity Ninja, Addiction Recovery Advocate, and CFS Recovery Mentor; specializes in reducing stress and anxiety for clients with ADHD and CFS. 25 years as a Simplicity Strategist in her own life has freed up space to enjoy life as a self-employed coach. A Certificate in Professional Coaching Practice in 2008 and has been a member of the International Coaching Federation (ICF) for 13 years.

Amanda was born in Scotland to Welsh parents and lived in East Yorkshire, England, and considers herself to be truly British. She loves lifelong learning, nature, and laughing until it hurts. Her motto to live by is 'Always leave people better than you found them.' (Marvin J. Ashton). She aims to educate the world on CFS and how it can be overcome, bringing hope to others who struggle.

Email: amanda.tremlett@hotmail.com
LinkedIn: www.linkedin.com/in/amanda-tremlett-dunn-023a3b172

-WW→

Tracey Vella

PART A

Who are you without your stories?

This was the day before I started to discover myself, and way before I learned that it doesn't matter who 'I was,' but more importantly, who 'I am'! Two decades before saying goodbye to who, and what, no longer aligned with my highest good - sitting in the shadows of negative mind programming. That night, everything changed, for everyone, and new stories developed. OH, imagine what I could have told my teenage self-back then from the energy space I now reside in!

It was a Thursday afternoon; I'd arrived home from school and made my way to my bedroom as I usually did. I flipped the page of my "inspirational" quotation calendar, which read – QUIT. I was in a good mood and was looking forward to going to bed that night, and to my parent's surprise, I went to have dinner with them at the table, something I had become estranged from. My Dad went to bed early, and my Mum was waiting to go to work. It was the 29th of July 1999, I was in grade 11, sweet 16, and yes, I'd been kissed. I seemed to have been in trouble a lot or not quite able to live up to expectations from a perfectionist parent who liked everything in a very particular way, not allowing to find or express myself nor show real emotion, to which I'd learnt to nervously close myself off, only to be told to "snap out of it".

"MUM!!!!". She was interrupted by me yelling in a muffled, panicked tone, followed by vomiting. It was now 2 am, and Mum had arrived home from work and went for a shower.

"Get up and run to the toilet," She yelled, thinking I was sick.

"I'm SO sorry, Mum" With more sounds of choking and vomiting, she came running. "What are you sorry for? What is wrong?" she replied.

In a low tone and slurred voice, I told her to look in my top drawer. She opened my dresser drawer to find it full of empty Panadol and Nurofen packets and a cocktail of drugs I had taken from the medicine cabinet. She turned around to see a note written on the mirror.

I'm sorry, Mum and Dad; I love you both.

The calendar inserts confirming, it was time to QUIT. Mum became numb. Dad came in to see what the commotion was. He quickly jumped into action, rushing me to the car to take me to the hospital, where the doctors were waiting for us. It was a blur. I remember vomiting multiple times and looking up to see a grade 12'er from school staring straight back at me, staring, judging. I woke up thinking this was not part of the plan; I was looking forward to going to bed and never waking up again.

The journey of my negative programming and conditioning.

I grew up in what seemed an average everyday working-class household. I was the youngest of 3. My parents were still together and very much each other's best friends. We lived on a sugar-cane farm amongst extended family, I went to a Catholic School, and we typically went to Church on a Saturday night - the makings of a conservative family.

Though from an early age, I always felt like the odd one out, being a sensitive kid emotionally and spiritually, the *black sheep of the family* is what came to my mind. Looking back, I was a truth seeker, on a search for something deeper, a change maker of years of programming, yet I was labelled as a difficult child, a stubborn little *witch/bitch*, being shut down like a Jack in the Box, I seemed to have been in trouble a lot or not quite able to live up to expectations from a perfectionist parent who liked everything in a very particular way, not allowing to find or express myself nor show real emotion, to which I'd learn to nervously close myself off, only to be told to "snap out of it".

I was a healthy child early on, though I did have a few illnesses growing up. Health is now a significant focus in my life - Natural ways of health.

I had ear problems at an early age, needing grommets. I contracted meningitis at 8, my adenoids were removed at 9, and at 11, I was diagnosed with Scoliosis, a curvature of the spine that would shape and eventually reshape my world. I feel a sense of solid emotions rising while reflecting on all this from my past. I think this has always sat there in the darker recesses of my mind, but I never really let myself FEEL it again in a cathartic way. I now feel a little overwhelmed as I write. *Do I want to go there*? I question myself, YES, I do. This needs to be told as I KNOW so many others go through this and keep it hidden from the world. You are not alone!

When I stopped growing, I no longer required bracing, and the curvature in my spine was measured at 27 degrees. Scoliosis never stopped me from doing the things I loved. I water-skied and played a lot of netball, being fit and healthy, until one day, I wasn't. Future pinched nerves, no doubt stemming from all of this; if I knew then the pain management and blood flow benefits of my current Ice bathing practices, maybe things would have been different for me.

I was 14 when I became sexually active. Having a catholic upbringing, the day I lost my virginity, I also felt I lost my dignity and respect. At 15, I was taken advantage of sexually on 2 separate occasions; I had locked these events deep in my memory, as I was ashamed and did not have the support I needed, and I felt I was to blame. I became bulimic, and this was the start of teenage drinking and drugs, a downward spiral of giving up and becoming a wayward teenager.

I guess you could say that my outbursts were a cry for help. A fitting help that never came.

During school I did not receive learning support, or guidance that I probably needed. Instead, I was classed as *lazy*, deemed as trouble, and labelled 'Brendan Vella's little sister,' having a teacher lecture me on how I would account for nothing and become a *no-hoper just like my brother*. I was then made a comparison to my sister with comments like, "Why can't you be more like your sister?" She was the goody-two-shoes-people-pleaser of the family. I was not academic at school and was asked to leave after grade 10 for receiving an unsatisfactory red behaviour card. When I changed schools in grade 11, I was confused and lost, lacked self-confidence and self-esteem, had no belief in myself nor direction in life, developed anxiety; and my mum had been recording a depression that would start around May and go through the winter. This is not a blame game, instead, as I mentioned above, it is how I started conditioning myself. None of us realise the impact of our actions or words might have on ourselves and others at the time, that impact made an imprint in how I viewed myself and how my unconscious would present later in life, with stories from childhood and negativity being deeply ingrained into my belief systems, I'd learnt to beat myself up for not being good enough, and became haunted by those "you are statements".

Through Yoga and Breath-work, I now have a 'return to self-energy,' and now I feel honoured I can BE that support to others I never had access to during my formative and traumatic years. I never received help as I did not look at the above as trauma; trauma was for the kids with a rough home life, living in poverty, or domestic violence. Instead, I had parents who tried their hardest and gave us what we needed. So, my learned behaviour was to beat myself up, *'What is wrong with me'?*

After my suicide attempt, I took time off school to recover. My mum's friend had given me a book called 'You Can Heal Your Life' by Louise Hay. I read it, but it was too much for my understanding. I was holding Anger and other emotions with no names. I doused the book in methylated spirits to try to burn it, but the book wouldn't burn, I took it as a sign and eventually re-read it. This was the start of my awakening journey.

I returned to grade 12, where I felt like I had a fresh start, however, it wasn't long before I would sabotage everything for myself again.

294

I fell pregnant. Although I had my Mums support, I didn't hesitate to have an abortion, I was not ready to be a teenage Mum. Not long after the abortion, a trail of disasters determined my mental state, and my boyfriend was involved in a car accident leaving him with head injuries. I decided that life was all too much for me. Looking for a different escape, I decided to run away with a guy I barely knew, all whilst my friends were doing their debutante. We camped on the banks of the Murray River; fruit picking was quite blissful, and something had changed in me; I wasn't reminded of who I was anymore, being away from everything I knew, the looks of sympathy, the guilt that reflected on me, the sadness from those who weren't sure how to treat me, and the shame and embarrassment I brought to my family.

While on the Murray River, I became connected to a deeper part of who I was. Being amongst nature and wildlife, everything spoke to me. I could feel the plants and the animals, an energy vibration from the earth. We swam in the cold river every day, and I felt so alive; I think these memory sensations flow back into my mind and body as I now slip into my Ice Bath.

This Murray experience was the moment that I became a vegan and felt for Mother Earth on a deep level. I found a passion I had never felt before, becoming obsessed with saving the earth and animals. Unfortunately, I was not in the right company to embark on my new passions. Instead, I was introduced to harder drugs and escaped even more. Thankfully, I felt there were always earth angels watching out for me, times when I knew God had intervened in what could have been serious or life-damaging events.

I returned home to celebrate my 18th birthday. Still on a quest to discover who I was and escape the triggers of family, I managed to find myself in negative relationships, more downward spirals of drugs, only this time domestic violence, heartache as well as adding trouble and stress caused to my family. After a couple of years of being lost and directionless, I left the scene and returned home, learning **you are not only what you eat, but you are also who you hang out with.**

Coming home to myself.

After a long dark winter, I had locked myself away from a cruel world that I had experienced. I gained strength and could feel life returning. I attended youth programs to return to work and joined Green Corps, where I received guidance for the future. With the gain of control after the struggle of another Winter, I realised I might be able to control the temperature in my life. I remembered what I loved doing and investigated what jobs would be adrenaline-fuelling, so as I could travel an endless summer. I discovered an Outdoor Recreation course in Cairns, which I applied for and was accepted.

Though, my sabotage seemed to be on an automated self-destruct cycle, as soon as I realised some sort of happiness, I would find a way to mess it up again, this time through more recreational drugs, and another pregnancy.

After already having an abortion and undergoing surgeries for vaginal issues, the Dr had warned me that 'if I ever wanted kids, I was to think about having them before the age of 25, as it was unlikely I would fall pregnant again.' With that information, I was convinced to keep the baby. My family was supportive; however, they were preparing to raise the baby, saying that the baby would either make or break me.

I had turned 21 and gave birth to my first-born son – Tijhe. I took motherhood into my stride, and to everyone else's surprise, he had saved my life, however, I felt that my dreams were squashed, a kind of entrapment.

I was stuck at home raising a baby on my own, second best to drugs and gambling. I was a good mum, though I was living in a state of stress, raising the baby through emotional abuse, constant fighting, and worry. I suffered silently with a deeply rooted depression growing deeper, stemming from my past, my mistakes, feeling like I wasn't enough, and my inability to live my dreams. I grew bitter and twisted, emotionally and physically, and my scoliosis worsened over time. The curve had gone from 27 to 37 degrees, with a new curve and rotation that developed in my lumbar spine, causing daily chronic pain, which I had become accustomed to.

After my suicide attempt, I detested pharmaceuticals.

Though I didn't quite know how to deal with my depression, I would ask the doctors for blood tests stating that I was not depressed, but I felt something was not functioning correctly in my body. He would always respond with, "It's all in your head; here is a script for anti-depressants," or he would offer pain medications. *All in my head*. I cried and pleaded that I wasn't depressed, with that ingrained belief that I had nothing to be depressed about and that my body felt like it was failing me— programming *manifestations*.

Life went on, and I got through it drug and medication-free but not mentally and physically pain-free.

Still unaware of this programming, I unconsciously created many dramas and self-sabotage, victimising myself and not allowing myself to be truly happy or feel deserving and worthy of happiness. I carried the blame around. I would sabotage relationships, friendships, and jobs feeling like I wasn't good enough, or I had the unconscious belief that it would be taken away from me.

I was 25 when I met my current partner, who had brought some fun and excitement back into my life. I didn't want the old habits to set back in, but they did. I came to a point where enough was enough. It was taking me a lot longer to recover. My hormones were so out of sync, my depressive emotional states and anxiety worsened, and I was not liking the person I was becoming. I had left Tijhe's dad for this very thing, so I gave Jonno an ultimatum to come into my world or leave it. To my surprise, he chose us!

-ᴡᴡᐳ

Tracey Vella

PART B

Adventure-Seeking Yogi

'Nothing changes if nothing changes' - The reprogramming.

A negative mindset is full of paranoia, believing that my past would continue along old processes and that what happened to me previously would repeat itself on autopilot. I thought no one loved me and I wasn't worthy of love, as love meant being hurt *in my head and my heart*, being cheated on, and being abused emotionally and physically.

I never allowed myself to be enough for Jonno. My stories were so loud inside my head, and on repeat. My defences were always switched on. My mental health quickly deteriorated, and my physical health worsened.

Jonno and I went on to have 2 more babies, Bodhi and Kohve, who were close in age at 15 months apart. It was after watching the health of our then 2-year-old decline that shaped our health journey. (This is a whole other story- save that for the next book!)

Bodhi changed our life; through his stomach issues, we learned all about gut health. We changed our diets to assist his, although this made a difference, I was never supported by my outer family, again the constant comments and lack of understanding; once again I was not shown the support to be able to trust in myself, nor the respect in our newfound lifestyle choices. I found it easier to distance myself from my family, being shut down from their limited views made it hard to be around.

After learning of Bodhi's stomach sensitivities, I, too, was going through similar health challenges, being tested for what the Doctors thought to be Crohn's or Coeliac disease, however tests couldn't confirm as I was already living a gluten free diet and I wasn't prepared to make myself sick for a piece of paper.

I was diagnosed with an autoimmune disease, Hypothyroidism, Fibromyalgia, and Premenstrual Dysphoric Disorder, PMDD. The Winters would continue to affect me, feeling depressed and not coping with raising 3 children with a partner that had to work away.

Backward and forward to the doctors for answers, never receiving a reason for these diagnoses nor how I could treat them naturally or learn of the root cause, I eventually gave up on the Orthodox medical system and turned to Natural Therapies, which my Naturopath took one look at my symptoms and told me I had Liver problems, not surprisingly after everything I had put my liver through. My gut health was also destroyed by my Bulimia, and I learned I wasn't absorbing nutrients nor making Hydrochloric acids in my stomach to have everything in good working order.

Through my many complexities, I was inspired to learn more about the body. I wasn't able to complete Naturopathy online, so I embarked on a Diploma of Massage Therapy, aiming to help people with their physical ailments and using massage as a steppingstone to continue studying more natural therapies

During this time, the stress of studying and finding time for family was difficult and my emotions were playing havoc. I found myself dancing with the old programming of taking my life. I broke down to Jonno, I felt I could not do this "Mum Life' or another Winter again.

"We need to make a major change," I cried. He agreed. We boarded the escape train and in 2015, we decided to pack up our house and go travelling.

During our travels, the pain in my body became severe. I was pinching a nerve in my pelvis, burning a hole down the front of my leg. We were at a market in Melany where I was limping around with tears falling from the pain. I met a man working there whom I was guided to chat with. Not having much faith in market practitioners, I asked him who I could see in town, someone with more knowledge than a man at a market. (Placing that judgement, criticism, and lack of trust onto him from my family conditioning. Interesting!)

I soon learned he would be the turning point in my life.

He told me to come and see him in his home, he wasn't even going to charge me, he just wanted to help me. He worked on my body for 3 hours, releasing pain and trauma that I learned was stored in my body from years of conditioning. He also suggested that I try Yoga. A week after my initial appointment with him, my world changed. My vision was crystal clear, everything shimmered, the colours were crisp, and the fog inside my head had released, as did the pain. He also told me that 'my younger self couldn't hurt me anymore.' What did this mean? It was at this point I was reawakened, to go against the grain of society to find my way in a deeply indoctrinated world. This was the start of changing my programming and the many years of memorised patterns. I was now Evolving.

I had finished my certificate 4 in Massage Therapy and decided to learn more about this newfound modality - Ortho Bionomy.

My real love for learning started when I began to help people with their pain and health journeys.

We settled in Airlie Beach, where I would start attending regular Yoga classes. At first, I felt so embarrassed, I had trouble touching my knees, never mind my toes. My mind was telling me to quit, as that's what I did with most things I couldn't do, however intuition was telling me to continue. I had little belief in the benefits of Yoga, after being told for so long that you won't be able to change your body, but the day I touched my toes, my mind was set, Yoga was life changing. This was huge, I had never been able to touch my toes, even as a child. I continued with classes, which I believe was helping me build resilience to the stress of having two young children as well as one pre-teen. I was desperate to learn.

After attending a few classes, the owner learning I was a Massage Therapist and offered me a job in the attached Day Spa. I continued my Yoga practice, which she then encouraged me to do my yoga teacher training. Never would I have thought I could become a Yoga teacher; I had zero confidence in public speaking and disliked being the centre of attention, I was far too judgmental and critical of myself to be put under that kind of pressure. However, I wanted to deepen my own practice and learn more about the body mechanics and principles of Yoga, to engage in a deeper meaning to life. It was at this point, something shifted; someone believed in me, a game changer.

Teaching Yoga has brought many like-minded people into our lives, confirming that we were not crazy with the health path we were on, it was also comforting to not have to justify our actions and diets anymore, instead surrounded by people who had similar stories.

After 9 months, we moved back to Mackay and into our old house. The house held the energy of frustration and being on an extremely busy road with noisy industrial areas behind us and domestic violence next door. I found myself spiralling backward, recognizing my old patterns emerging, only this time the difference was that I had my Yoga in my toolbox and started my own Massage Studio.

NO WAY - NOT AGAIN!

After a healthier lifestyle, and trying many therapies, including Counselling, Psychology, Kinesiology, Chiropractic, Reiki, Healers, Nutritional Therapy, Hormone Suppositories, Acupuncture, Sound Therapy, Shamanic healing, Rapid Eye Movement for PTSD, Psychotherapy, Psychosomatic Therapy, Winter still took its grip on me.

I felt defeated and went searching mainstream mental health for answers.

Whilst in the waiting room, I talked myself into leaving, remembering how this place did me no favours in my youth. The social worker caught me walking out and convinced me to have a chat. As we sat down, he asked, "Tell me about yourself, as your Aura does not speak of mental illness to me". He had my attention. He asked what I did for fitness, as I looked fit and healthy, and my body language was not of the typically depressed people. I explained to him that I had been doing Yoga. "How much?" he asked, "At least 5 to 6 times a week," I responded. "Ah, Ha, sounds to me like you are releasing a lot of stored traumas from your body, and your mind is trying to intellectualise it." He told me to keep doing Yoga and just to let go. This was the first time I had heard of Yoga achieving this - releasing our issues from our tissues. *Issues from our Tissues.* Love this!

From Louise Hay and other body language books, I understood our emotional traumas were stored manifesting in our physical body as illness and disease, though I never knew how to release the trauma, instead I would become resentful when learning the possible root causes which resonated from my childhood wounds.

I began seeing a mind coach in 2015, who I still see today, and she assisted me on many levels, more than psychology ever did, teaching me about the brain and a technique called Emotional Freedom Technique or Tapping, (Tapping). She helped me understand that trauma was trauma, no matter how big or small, not to be so hard on myself, to stop judging myself so harshly and to start to believe in myself.

However, the next Winter came around, and although they were becoming shorter, I still suffered. I stumbled across a book by Joe Dispenza 'Breaking the Habit of Being Yourself', (published by Hay House Inc, 2013). This was another pivotal point in my life, diving deep into all Dispenza's work, learning all about the mind and how it influences our physical health. Symptoms began easing, but nothing yet broke through the depression.

2018 I learned of the Medical Medium, and 2019 I went through an intensive heavy metals detox. I strongly believed this would be the icing on the cake, together with Joe Dispenza's work, the tapping, Yoga, and clean eating. I would say goodbye to my seasonal affective disorder once and for all. But 2020's Winter has arrived, and I fell deeper than the year before.

I was DONE! *Why this crazy cycle when I've done so much work on myself?*

2020, a confusing and stressful time for all of us, Seasonal Affective Disorder was debilitating, so much so that I was planning to leave my family. I'd believed that Jonno and the kids would be better off without me, and my "drama", I feared instilling the same traumas and negativity as I felt as a child onto my own. I became too hard on myself, giving up all that I loved, believing nothing worked. I sat in heavy introspection of self-blame for past traumas, holding myself accountable for my negative personality traits and taking responsibility for the pain and suffering I caused myself and my family, something most people avoid. I sat in the depths of the "Dark Night of the Soul" which was a blessing in disguise, I let go of toxic relationships and handed control and responsibility over to my partner.

Jonno became so scared of losing me, began his search for strength and personal development. He knew he needed to change his ways and habits and step up. I had completely given up on myself and my family. I stopped doing what I loved in the belief that nothing was working, "this is who I am, and I am now accept it."

I would cry.

Nothing seemed to help, and I had thrown a lot of money into therapies that had promised would. Jonno loving me unconditionally through depression, anxiety, and all, would help change my unconscious programming. He never once said, "What is your problem now" which is what I had received from my family. Instead, he fought for our lives.

Jonno had stumbled across the Wim Hof Method. He tried the breathwork himself and felt a massive shift in his mental state. He then introduced it to me; I told him to "F**K OFF" and to stop trying to change me, that I had accepted my condition after 20-

plus years of living with it. He pleaded with me, breaking down, trying to get me to see that this wasn't who I was.

"Please, for all of us, just give it a go," He asked me to do it with him and not to read up about it until I felt the benefits.

Holding hope, we began the Wim Hof Breathwork. It took me on a profound journey; I growled, cried, laughed, and found peace. I truly profoundly EVOLVED on another plane of existence; *"how much do you want to change?* (You know the answer!)

I felt high again, remembering how much I loved that feeling.

I continued the breath work daily. Jonno suggested I read Wim Hof's book, 'The Wim Hof Method - Activate your full Human Potential' (Wim Hof, 2020, Sounds True Publishers). We then started the cold-water therapy. The book grabbed me instantly and affected me deeply, I learned how Wim Hof lost his wife to suicide; she kissed their 4 children goodbye before jumping off an 8-story building in front of them. This is why Jonno resonated so profoundly with this method. After losing the love of his life to suicide, his pain was so deep that one day he jumped into an ice-cold lake having nothing to focus on but his breath and survival. He earned that together, the cold and his breath would take away his mental anguish. Jonno felt the same and was desperate for me to find it too, as this would not be our fate.

I finished his book, then introduced cold showers in May. This was hard as I have always hated the cold; whenever I hesitated, I would ask myself - "how much do you want to change?" We started with 15 seconds a week, eventually increasing weekly until I could do 2 minutes. That year, the Winter did not come, my depression was non-existent. I couldn't believe it; I even went looking for it. In August, we plunged into our first Ice bath. I stepped out feeling so alive, yet I cried; it was a cry of gratitude, I felt as though I witnessed my own funeral, the death of my old self. My chemistry and physiology were changed, and I knew this was the golden ticket. *This was it!*

I found out it's not something you do once, and you're fixed; it has become a practice that we have incorporated into our everyday lives. During the breathwork, I started incorporating all of the techniques I had learned, using the breath holds as a meditation time to reprogram my mind. I started with "I am loved, loving and lovable," "I love and accept myself," to "I am accepting and accepted." Those became my mantras for months.

I allowed my traumas to come up, still working through them with the emotional freedom technique, becoming much easier to shift, not affecting me or causing too much introspection like it once had. I forgave myself and others. The day I forgave my firstborn's dad out loud to him changed everything for me; that deeply ingrained trauma was healed, taking away all the trauma and anxiety I once held, taking back my power to no longer be a victim of my past and to own and be responsible for the part I played.

I went through these 4 steps with everything that had caused me big trauma.

1- Forgiving myself for whatever role I had played in the situation.

2- Forgiving others for their role in hurting me, finding compassion for where they came from.

3- Giving other people permission to forgive me, is a big one, as when we hold ourselves in self-hatred, as I did for many years, we don't feel worthy of people's forgiveness.

4- And finally, asking God for forgiveness for the part I played, believing in God or not, this felt like a major part, as you allow a source much greater than you to show you unconditional love, and it is this love and vibration that we embody.

After these deep shifts in consciousness of mind, body and spirit, life has been an uphill journey from here. I continued with my Yoga daily, eventually having my body pain go from a constant 8/10 down to 1- 2/10. I was curious to see what the curve in my spine measured after being told it would only deteriorate, degenerate and worsen.

In 2021 upon investigation, we compared X-rays from 2017 to the current one, to our surprise, I had corrected the curve in my lumbar spine, rotating it back to normal. I had also changed the degree of the curve in my mid-thoracic spine from 37 degrees to a 34-degree curvature.

I was stoked, having proved medical professionals wrong, as I was always told there was nothing I could do, my spine would only continue to degenerate and compress.

This was the start of my believing in what I do, as I had physical proof! When I asked the chiropractor if it could get any better, he responded – "textbook no, but keep doing what you're doing."

Being out of pain, and depression and no longer a victim to my ailments, I started my Yoga business, Adventure Seeking Yogi in 2021, taking my guests on retreats purposely during Winter, inviting the Winter in. I broke through my comfort zones achieving my versions of impossible from attaining my commercial boat licence and working on many boats, sailing up and down the QLD coastline, to meeting many amazing people.

Finding my breath, practising Yoga and starting the ice baths has given me my life back, healing physically, mentally, emotionally and spiritually, no longer suffering the conditions once diagnosed with, all without medical intervention. Unfortunately, this was no quick fix, but a journey that would take me to the depths of my mind, body and soul, to heal deeply ingrained traumas, to find forgiveness, to sit in my shadows and to reprogram my mind. I have learnt boundaries, saying goodbye to who and what no longer aligns to my highest good, during my solitude, I found my true tribe.

Sure, I still have struggles, but I am more resilient and able to work through struggles with a clear mind. A mind that is no longer trapped in survival mode from stress and anxiety but has switched over into a new state, escaping the constant stressful state that I once lived in, I have now been able to study methods of what has helped me, to be able to work with people in one on one or group session of yoga, breathwork and ice baths, to aid in their health and wellness desires, assisting them in making positive changes for quality of life, so they can be the best version of themselves, for themselves and their families.

I no longer beat myself up (as harshly) and have learned that it doesn't matter about Who I was, what it matters is Who I am. It's OK to step outside of who you know and unlearn what you have been programmed to believe, to find what fits you, not what fits the mould of family and mainstream societal conditioning. I evolve daily, I blog, I travel, I sail, I breathe, I love, and I live.

People have asked me about 'end results', I don't have any 'end results' as such. My vision is to simply EVOLVE with health and all those who resonate with my energy and whom I work with, EVOLVING via Yoga, Connection and my New Rules of Wellness.

That night in July 1999 when everything changed for everyone, I didn't know it then, but new stories developed, A new dance to dance. Through that experience, I've discovered myself on a deeper plane. Don't let yourself become defeated, who are you or who can you become without your stories?

About the Author

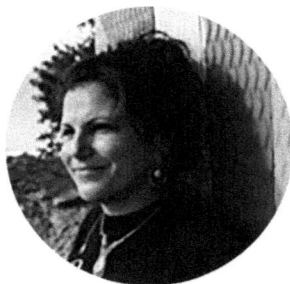

Tracey Vella is an Adventure Seeking Yogi who owns and runs her business of the same title, assisting others to hold the space for themselves and their own growth through life stresses, past health crises, and traumas.

She avidly enjoys Breathwork, Yoga, and Ice Baths as therapeutic tools. She directly communicates the energy with 'issues from our body's tissues', re-programming biology and thinking patterns. She knows with clarity this is the key to changing lives and loves all things Natural and "Alternative" Therapies. Through these methods, she got her life back, and now she can take people on adventures to inspire others to take their life back too.

Tracey enjoys quiet cups of tea in nature from her Earthenware 'HOPE' mug and a claw-footed bath in a paddock, and you may well find her at the beach or in their caravan, or on a Sailing vessel out at sea, quietly thriving.

She evolves, blogs, basks, travels, breathes, loves, and LIVES daily.

Tracey's Message: Your future is unknown, and so is your potential.

Website: www.adventureseekingyogi.com
Facebook: https://www.facebook.com/Adventureseekingyogi
Email: traceyv83@live.com

-⌇⌇⌇→

Barb Whitfield

Be Well Be Happy

Let's face it; sometimes life gets hard; we all need to be heard, feel supported, and have trust in someone. I hold space. *What is that?* I hear you think. Some of my Wellness family, I call every single person that has ever had a session with me a part of my wellness family. Call me "The calmness in the chaos of life." I assist you in finding your space, inner calmness, and resilience, so you can breathe long and deep again and enjoy your life to the fullest, whatever that may look like for you. I hold space for you.

People I meet often ask me, *"What do you do?"* I answer: *"I assist and support individuals, just like you, to live their life to the fullest, achieve their goals no matter how big or small, to be well and happy."*

Sometimes a simple breath technique taught to someone with inconsistent and broken sleep can assist with their sleep soundness and improve their life. Being continually tired lowers your immunity and significantly stresses your mental wellness. A solid and sound sleep boosts your health and happiness and can put a bounce in your step again.

Other times I support individuals that have cancer or chronic illness. A simple meditation and relaxation technique can give a person space to be and time to accept where they are in life so they can fulfill and achieve what makes them happy.

When I have my first session with someone, I see their body language, how they sit, walk, how they breathe, and whether the light in their eyes is bright. All these things leap out at me and tell me a story.

It all depends on an individual's story, and we all have a story to tell; it just depends on who is listening and if it's being heard. I listen deeply and consciously. I hear unspoken words.

Simply put, I'm a Life Doula.

Sometimes I only see an individual once as that's all they need, and others regularly. It depends on the person's needs. The best thing is I'm always here to assist. ☺

I was given a piece of very useful advice a very long time ago that I like to live by.

Always accept what is and build on the positive.

I'd love to share some of my wellness family journeys. I hope you enjoy reading them as much as I feel blessed and honored to be a part of their story.

Emily's Journey

Emily came to see me as she was anxious all the time, and this was affecting her sleep. She hadn't had a good night's sleep for a very long time and felt lethargic and depressed. Getting out of bed and going to work had become a massive struggle as she had no energy or vitality. Emily said she was crying at the drop of a hat, and the minor thing seemed to upset her.

She had seen her doctor for a checkup, and her blood tests had returned normal. However, he was concerned that her blood pressure was higher than usual and she had gained weight. He had placed her on medication to control her high blood pressure.

A large part of what I do is chat and observe in my sessions. I learn much more about a person's life and story over a conversation, deep listening, and observation than any document can tell me.

After a while, Emily told me that her corporate job didn't inspire her, her employer seemed to expect too much from her, and she felt underappreciated.

She was sick of feeling tired, washed out, having no energy, and feeling off-color. The joy of her life had been replaced with unhappiness. Emily said she felt unwell physically and mentally.

Emily also shared that she was married, had adult children that had all flown the coup, and was an internationally qualified yoga teacher. She practiced yoga and meditation daily and ate a nutritious diet.

After listening to Emily and her story, I asked her how I could assist her. She simply said she wanted to be happy and enjoy her life again. I inquired if she would be open to going for a special kind of walk each day. She said she would try anything to feel like her old self again.

Research shows that walking is an easy weight-bearing exercise that can be adapted to suit everyone; it reduces the risk of breast cancer, eases joint pain, improves bone density, encourages weight loss, boosts immune function, reduces blood pressure, and improves heart and mental health.

Deep breathing while walking can reduce menopause systems in 80% of females.

I explained to Emily that breath walk sessions are inclusive for all and can be adapted for anybody, any age, and any ability. They include walking and breathing patterns, sound, and with finger magic. There are 5 components to a Breath Walk session, warmup, check-in with self, vitality section, deep relaxation, and meditation. Breath Walks can take 30 minutes to an hour, depending on which one you do.

Breath Walk sessions assist you in having improved energy and vitality, elevate your mental clarity and enhance your wellness and well-being. The body, mind, and spirit work together when you learn to breathe and walk consciously.

There are 20 breath walks programs; each session is designed to have a specific effect.   For example, one is for a Clear Mind for people who want to reduce mental clutter. Another 1 is for those wanting to increase their vitality, named Quick Start Energy Booster.

After discussing with Emily which walk would be the most beneficial for her, we decided on the breath walk for Simple Anxiety to Inner Calm for her to do daily for 40 days. We both felt that this walk would assist and support her in improving her well-being and wellness.

Emily started her session with a slow, easy warmup of breathing and slow, gentle body movements to prepare the body and mind for the rest of the program. She began walking gently, checking in with herself about her feelings. The next part of this walk involved simply coordinating breathing segments and walking. This is the vitality section. It uses finger magic. (I love this term!) This is simply fingers touching each other in time with the breathing and walking. Gradually, Emily slowed the pace, allowing her senses to expand as she gathered her energy from her Breath Walk. This walk finishes sitting and doing a guided sensory breath meditation.

I checked in with Emily every few weeks to see how she felt. She had taken herself through the session every day and started to notice after only 2 weeks that her anxiety levels were decreasing, and she was feeling better about herself. Mentally she felt more robust and less emotional. This encouraged her to keep doing it. After 4 weeks, Emily noticed that her energy had returned, and she had a bounce in her step again.

After 70 days of doing her daily session (even in the rain), she returned to her doctor to check her blood pressure, which had been slowly rising before she came to see me. Her doctor was amazed as her blood pressure had significantly lowered, she was smiling, and some weight had disappeared. Her doctor asked what she had been doing and was told *a Breath Walk*. Her doctor said to *keep doing it*!!!

At the time of writing this, it has been over 200 days since Emily started her journey back to finding herself happy and well again. She has caught every day of her walk. She even did her sessions on a holiday cruise with her family and other short breaks away. Every time I see her, a beautiful smile beams from her face, and I feel blessed to have assisted and supported her. Emily is aiming to continue her daily practice for 1000 days. I am sure that she will complete it.

As a certified yoga teacher, Emily has now completed the training in How to Teach a Breath Walk; in time, she will teach Breath Walk sessions to others seeking to improve their well-being and wellness.

Ricks Life

Rick contacted me via my webpage about seeing me. As he lived on the other side of Australia, I suggested we meet via Zoom. Zoom is a platform that can be used on a phone, laptop, or handheld device so people can see, talk, and hear each other in real-time. We set up a time and date that worked for him, and as he had never used Zoom before, I telephoned him before our first session and talked him through the easy setup.

I asked Rick how I could assist him, and he explained that he was a full-time carer for his wife, who had cancer, and he wanted to find himself again. I asked him what he meant by *finding himself again*. Rick shared that he felt he had lost his identity, no longer had a career, and wasn't a husband, lover, or friend to his wife; he was a carer. He and his wife didn't have anything they could do together anymore due to her decline in health. His days were consumed with her pain medications, cooking nutritious broths for his wife, keeping her as comfortable as he could, phone calls, and doctor and nurse visits. He was the cleaner, the bottlewasher, everything. He felt ashamed that he felt this way; he was the one that was supposed to keep it all together. He loved his wife and wanted to be with her, mainly because their time was limited.

I neutrally listened with no judgment and quietly asked if he felt overwhelmed; he looked down and hesitated for a moment; I explained that what we discussed stayed private and confidential with me. Rick looked up at me; he said he felt like he was sinking and was so overwhelmed that he was having trouble breathing. His voice sounded shaky, he kept swallowing, and I noticed his hands trembling. His breathing was erratic.

Rick shared that he couldn't talk to his family about this as he was sure they would judge him for not being a man and caring for everything. The tears started to trickle down Rick's face as he started to cry, he put his face in his hands, and I held space for him. I sat there, not saying a word.

Having someone to be there and listen to you and just be there can be a huge relief and life-changing.

When no more tears were to shed, I asked Rick how he felt. He said, relieved as a huge burden had just been lifted from his shoulders, and it was good to talk to me without the fear of judgment. He said that he had not cried for a long time, especially not since his wife's diagnosis or illness. Rick was feeling unburdened with his release of emotion and tears.

Studies have shown that crying is suitable for your physical and mental health. It can be an essential safety value as bottling up emotions and keeping everything inside of you can lead to a lower immune system, increased blood pressure, and cardiovascular disease.

We discussed what was happening with him being the carer for his wife and if he was receiving any support looking after her. Rick explained that he would inquire about getting respite care for a couple of hours a week. He had been putting it off as he didn't want to look like he wasn't coping. I assured him it was good for his physical and mental health to ask for assistance and have some time off.

I asked Rick if he was open to doing some daily breath work as this would assist him in managing his stress, increase his ability to cope, and hopefully not become so overwhelmed again. He thought that would be achievable as he could do it when his wife was asleep.

Our bodies react to life events as they unfold. Stress, especially, can take its toll on our bodies physically and mentally. It can affect a person's body, thoughts, feelings, and behavior. Stress also affects the nervous system and the hormonal reactions in a person's body.

Stress and feeling overwhelmed can be assisted with breath work and relaxation techniques.

I explained to Rick that Long Deep Breathing (LDB) was easy to do, and it worked by relaxing and calming the body due to its influence on the parasympathetic nervous system. This part of the nervous system allows us to experience calmness. LDB mainly involves the nose, chest area (lungs and ribs), belly, and diaphragm to inhale and exhale fully. It can be down sitting or lying down.

As Rick was sitting on a chair, we decided to start here. I asked him to keep his spine tall and his feet flat on the floor. I asked if he felt comfortable closing his eyes, and he said yes and closed them. I requested that Rick notice his breathing flow and inhale and exhale slowly. While doing this, place one hand on his belly, just below the ribs, and the other on his chest. I coached Rick to take a slow, deep breath, inhaling slowly through his nose, paying attention as his belly swelled up under his hand, his ribs expanded, and his upper chest lifted. Then slowly release the breath through the nose, in reverse order, emptying the upper chest, ribcage, and belly like blowing up a balloon. The balloon fills up at the bottom, halfway, then top, and empties reversely.

While Rick continued breathing this way for several minutes, I noticed his breathing had become longer and had a slower rhythm. I asked him to inhale and suspend his breath, relax his hands and exhale when he was ready, and just sit to count his many blessings. He opened his eyes, and I asked him how he was feeling. He stated that he felt calmer, more balanced, and relaxed.

I suggested that Rick do several minutes of Long, Deep Breathing daily, and if he felt confident enough, he could teach his wife, and they could spend this time together.

I checked in with Rick 1 month later, as he had asked to see me monthly, and he seemed different. He smiled and explained that he had taught his wife the breath, and they had found their relationship had become close again as they shared quality time. It had brought a sense of togetherness and calmness to their home. I asked him if had found himself again, and he smiled and said yes, he was coping well and enjoying his time with his wife again. He had a sense of well-being and self-worth again. He then thanked me for being *The calmness in the chaos of life.*

When writing this, it has been 6 months since Rick first contacted me. He is still doing his breathing technique and feels that he can cope with whatever life brings.

Joy's Improvement

I've only seen Joy six times over a 3-month as she was highly motivated, did what I suggested daily, and quickly improved. She originally had called me after her doctor had given her my card and suggested she contact me to assist with her balance. As Joy got older, she noticed she seemed not as stable on her feet and mentioned it to her doctor. I went to Joy's house and chatted with her about her health and wellness, and I asked her what her goal was. She explained that she wanted to stay active and well to continue to enjoy her life living in her own home and return to her favorite pastime, ballroom dancing. She had stopped going dancing as she was afraid of falling in front of her friends. Joy said she was missing catching up with everyone and getting dressed up.

I taught Joy a couple of movements that would improve her balance. She was very surprised as they were simple and would only take about 10 minutes, 3 x times a day. At each visit, Joy improved, and I changed the movements to challenge her more. When I saw her last week (when writing this), she was progressing well with her balance and stability. I showed her how to progress the moments when she felt they were too easy. She had bought a new dress and planned to return to dancing in the next few weeks.

Joy wanted to continue her exercises independently as she was confident doing them. I reassured her that if she needed me again, to contact me.

I've always felt that I've been given a special gift to share with all that cross my path. Something given to me way before my birth, the eternal flame in my heart, tells me we are all connected and everything happens for a reason. The universe guides me where I need to be and brightens my light for those who may benefit from finding me.

I was 12 years old when my mother passed over; the week before, she told me, "Always *accept what is and build on the positive.*" This has been the guiding piece of light I've followed throughout my life.

Thank you for taking the time to read my chapter, I'd love to offer you a free Breath Work information sheet to assist sleep soundness and calmness. You will find my contact details in my bio.

Please reach out if you or a family member could benefit from seeing me. I would feel blessed and honored to assist you however I can—either face-to-face or via the simple technology of Zoom.

The first step can be the hardest.

Until our paths cross again, blessings and safe travels. Barb

About the Author

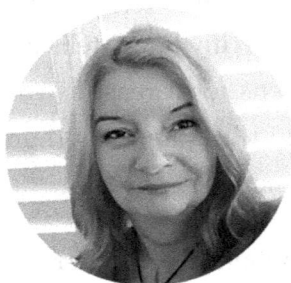

Barb Whitfield created and founded 'Be Well with Barb' over 35 years ago. She comes from a health science background that spans over 4 decades.

Barb is the designer of several national training programs, including 'It's Your Life Be Active,' 'Ageing with Vitality,' and 'Breath into Life.' Barb has received several national awards for her contributions to the health and wellness area, and she lectures nationally and internationally.

Her dream is to heal the world one person at a time. Being down to earth and an eternal optimist, she thinks outside the box, passionate about assisting individuals in finding their quiet calmness within.

Website: bewellwithbarb.com.au
Email: barb@bewellwithbarb.com.au
Facebook: https://www.facebook.com/bewellwithbarb